Hearing rehabilitation for deafened adults

A psychosocial approach

Dedication

In memory and honour of Raymond Hetu

Hearing rehabilitation for deafened adults

A psychosocial approach

Anthony Hogan, PhD
University of Sydney

W
WHURR PUBLISHERS
LONDON AND PHILADELPHIA

First published 2001 by
Whurr Publishers Ltd
19B Compton Terrace, London N1 2UN, England and
325 Chestnut Street, Philadelphia PA 19106, USA

British Library Cataloguing in Publication Data
A catalogue record for this book is available from the British Library.

ISBN: **978-1-86156-215-9**

Contents

Acknowledgements vii
Introduction xi

PART I Factors Impacting on the Psychosocial Predisposition of Clients with Hearing Loss 1

Chapter 1 3

A conceptual framework for a psychosocial approach to hearing rehabilitation

Chapter 2 24

The onset of deafness

Chapter 3 43

Carving out a space to act: acquired impairment and contested identity

PART II Addressing Psychosocial Issues within Rehabilitation Programmes for Deafened People 59

Chapter 4 61

Addressing everyday barriers to cochlear implantation

Chapter 5 72

Psychosocial approaches to hearing rehabilitation: it's a matter of process

Chapter 6 96

Engaging the client in a helping relationship
Anthony Hogan and Chris Code

Chapter 7 115

Structuring interventions

Chapter 8 131

Enhancing employment outcomes
Anthony Hogan, Lee Kethel, Kate White and Andrea Lynch

Chapter 9 139

The everyday benefits of cochlear implantation

PART III Psychosocial Rehabilitation Programmes 145

Chapter 10 147

A communication skills programme for people with acquired hearing loss

Appendix 199
References 201

PART IV Handouts (for photocopying) 211

Index 243

Acknowledgements

The research behind this book commenced in 1993 and was initially funded by a University of Wollongong Doctoral Scholarship in the Department of Public Health. In 1994 I was awarded a doctoral scholarship by the Department of Employment Education and Training in the Department of Sociology at Macquarie University. The study was also funded by a supplementary doctoral scholarship provided by Cochlear Ltd and administered by the respective universities.

The results of this study would not have been achieved without the support and direction of Professor Christine Ewan from the University of Wollongong, and Associate Professor Gary Dowsett and Dr Lyn Davis from Macquarie University. The Department of Sociology at Macquarie University became an intellectual home for me. In particular, the support of Dr Mitchell Dean, Dr Alan Taylor, Anne Barbato, Suzanne Anderson and Di Southwell (Research Librarian) is noted with thanks. At Cochlear Ltd, particular thanks go to Therese Kramer, Martha Follent, Nicki Lord, Sandra Pascuzzo, Debra Pannowitz and Albert Sorrell. I am grateful to Professor William Noble of the University of New England for introducing me to the Montreal model and for supporting my earlier work in this area.

To the co-ordinators and staff of the various branches of Better Hearing Australia, the differing cochlear implant clinics in Australia and New Zealand (with special thanks to Lee Kethel, Ellen Giles, Ellen McNeill, Karen Pedley, Emma Rushbrooke and Merril Stewart), and the Behavioural Epidemiology Unit, South Australian Health Commission, thank you for the support you have given me, for allowing me to use your facilities and for encouraging people to participate. Most specifically, thanks goes to everyone who agreed to participate in the research behind this text study, particularly Glenn Munnerley. I trust that I have been true to the stories you told me.

My wife Karen originally convinced me that I was capable of undertaking this project and has supported me in every way possible throughout it. No greater love than to live with someone through a doctoral thesis and then a book production! For parental support, Barbara and Paul, Max and Maria — I would not have made it without you.

Copyright acknowledgements

The Code-Müller Protocols questionnaire in Chapter 6 is reproduced with permission from Code and Müller (1992) *The Code-Müller Protocols: Assessing Perceptions of Psychosocial Adjustment to Aphasia and Related Disorders* (London: Whurr). The hearing and listening skills programme presented in Chapter 10 is adapted from the Hearing and Listening Skills Programme developed by Professors Louise Getty and Raymond Hetu of the University of Montreal and is reproduced with permission. In addition to the work the author carried out on the Montreal programme, further original contributions to the programme were made by Karen Pedley and Emma Rushbrooke. Jeanette Brazel assisted with the drawing of the Bar-B-Que exercise. Their contributions are also acknowledged and used with permission.

Exercises entitled *Responding to challenging situations* are adapted with permission from the original work of Christopher Lind. The original exercises were entitled 'Effective Communication – Getting what you want from conversation' and 'Effective Communication – responding to challenging situations' and were part of the Victorian Hear Service's Coping with Hearing Loss programme.

The Taoist relaxation exercise presented in the hearing and listening skills programme was originally published by Ken Cohen (1992) in the audiotape 'Taoist Healing Imagery – Traditional Chinese healing visualization', Sounds True Production, Boulder, CO, USA. The product is available through the Sounds True website, www.soundstrue.com

The restaurant exercise is from H. Kaplan, S. Bally, and C. Garrestson (1985) *Speechreading: A Way to Improve Understanding*, reproduced with the permission of Gallaudet University Press.

Chapter 3, 'Carving out a space to act', appeared as an original article in *Health* 2(1) 1998, and as a chapter in M. Corker and S. French (eds),

Disability Discourse (Open University, 1998). It is reproduced with permission.

The NLP exercise presented in the hearing and listening skills programme was based on original work by Andreas and Andreas (1994) and is reproduced with permission.

Parts of Chapter 9 originally appeared in Hogan (1997) 'Implant outcomes, towards a mixed methodology for evaluating the efficacy of adult cochlear implant programmes', *Disability and Rehabilitation*, Vol 19: 233–44, and are reproduced with permission.

Introduction

I first became aware of the need for specific rehabilitation services for Deafened adults during a community consultation I held in a small country town on the north coast of New South Wales, Australia, in 1989. At the time I was employed as the Manager of Community Services with the New South Wales Deaf Society. Technologies such as cochlear implants were then regarded as experimental and certainly were controversial. Hearing rehabilitation services, although established in some parts of the world, were barely established in Australia and to date are still quite thin on the ground. The consultation was held on a Saturday afternoon, in a drafty room, at the back of a servicemen's club. At this meeting I was confronted by the stark reality of what it was like for people, not simply to lose their hearing, but with the realities of what it was like to build a life as a Deafened person in a hearing world without adequate help, a useful technology, a support network or conceptual framework for understanding oneself in a new world.

Only a handful of people turned up to the consultation, yet what they had to say changed my life forever. They were basically older people who had lost their hearing over time. They had sought out every form of help they could find, and spent all they had on expensive hearing aids, but to no avail. They had been left to fare as best they could in the world without adequate assistance or support. Hearing loss had devastated their lives and left them on the margins of society as impoverished, isolated and broken people. I simply could not understand how these things had come to pass. Why did our society treat people like this? Why was there no help available for them? Why should hearing loss result in such marginalization? What could be done to change things? What particularly annoyed me was that I knew that this was not the way things had to be. I knew many Deafened people who were living out meaningful and empowered lives.

But what I was to later learn was that these few people were the exceptions. They had somehow accessed sufficient support and resources to carve out a reasonable life for themselves. Knowing that things could be otherwise, I was determined that something be done and this something set me on an odyssey that twelve years later has resulted in the writing of this book.

Much has changed since I held that first consultation so long ago. Cochlear implants and high gain hearing aids have come into their own as technologies that provide useful auditory input for many Deafened adults. Yet despite the media hype surrounding these so-called miracle technologies, most of the Deafened people I know still have very real problems managing difficult communication settings in everyday life. So while technologically things have improved, socially much has stayed the same. Certainly it would be good if the world sat up and started to treat Deafened people with the respect and consideration due to them. But this is not going to occur without a generational process of social change. In the mean time, Deafened people need to be equipped with the skills that will enable them to negotiate communicative life successfully in a hearing world, for this is where most of them want to be. Twelve years ago the Deafened people at the community consultation gave priority to two things – assistance with self-esteem, and aid in finding meaningful, paid employment. The detail provided in this book sets out to address these needs.

This book is intended to be used by people seeking to assist Deafened people and their partners to adjust to the disability they have acquired. I say 'they' because it is a shared experience, everyone's life changes when deafness enters a family. I would envisage that the text will be useful to professionals and consumer advocates working in hearing therapy services. Consumer feedback during the writing process suggests that many aspects of the text may also be useful to Deafened people themselves. As one person said to me, 'at last, someone has some idea of what it is we are going through'. Finally, I have found that my students in audiology, speech language pathology and rehabilitation counselling have found the materials to be accessible and practical in nature. Indeed, there is a dearth of material available in this field so I hope that this text will begin to fill some of this knowledge gap while stimulating others to go on to do future research in this field.

How to use this book

The overall purpose of this text is to provide the reader with a conceptual framework and description of skills required to successfully implement a basic psychosocial rehabilitation programme with clients with acquired hearing loss. The first nine chapters of the text seek to prepare the reader, at least conceptually, to engage with their clients in a meaningful and competent manner. Of course, life is the best teacher and it is my experience that once a level of academic competence has been achieved with the materials in this text, then one can move on to working with the materials and clients under supervision. Chapter 10 details a psychosocial rehabilitation programme.

Much of the work in this text centres on the experiences of people who lose all or most of their hearing. However, I have worked successfully on these materials with people with differing degrees of loss and various aetiologies. Overall I would say that people with acquired hearing loss have many experiences in common. The major difference is in the extent or degree of the experience, how hard, for example, it was to maintain family communication or to retain employment.

Structurally the text can be viewed in three phases. Part I (Chapters 1–3) is concerned with factors impacting on the psychosocial predisposition of clients with hearing loss. Part II (Chapters 4–9) is concerned with practical considerations to which the practitioner should give consideration in preparing to implement a psychosocial programme in his or her clinic. Part III (Chapter 10) is the rehabilitation programme itself.

The first three chapters seek to enable the reader to understand the personal and social issues confronting Deafened people. Adequate understanding of these materials is central to successful rehabilitation. Professionally experienced readers may be inclined to skip over this section, considering that they would be familiar with much of this material. This would be *ill-advised*. These introductory chapters take a sociological approach to hearing rehabilitation, seeking as they do to enable the reader to begin to understand why it is so difficult for Deafened people simply to tell other people that they are deaf. And why it is that society is so awful to Deafened people? The Surrealist artist, Joàn Miró, depicted this dilemma well in the landscape – *The Hare*. The story of the hare is one in which the central character lives in two worlds but is marginal to both.

The first chapter of this text lays out the social theory that underpins the social experience of marginality and then proceeds to detail the psychological consequences of such marginality. At this point a cautionary observation is made. This is a theoretical chapter that seeks to describe the landscape of experiences that Deafened people may encounter as they come to terms with their deafness. I do not, even for a moment, suggest that what I describe here is experienced by every or any Deafened person. It is for Deafened people to look into Miró's hare and to describe for themselves the consequences of deafness in their lives. For the reader, the chapter seeks to prepare you to listen to your clients with empathic understanding, to have some idea of what it may be like to walk a day in their shoes and to begin to appreciate just how difficult it might be to do the various things we ask of our clients in rehabilitation. For what we ask of them is actually to disrupt every social interaction that they engage in, to have people change the way they sit and stand, to alter the pace at which they speak and to restructure what they say. We actively encourage people to rearrange rooms, restaurants and the like and even suggest that people be told to shave off their beards. We are telling our clients to go out and change the world without for a moment taking into account the social capital that is at stake here, the differentials in social power between so-called able and disabled people, not to mention taken-for-granted social mores. We are in fact asking our clients to seriously risk further stigmatization in a society that cares little for those who do not readily fit in with our busy schedules. It is indeed hardly surprising that so many clients simply do not implement the strategies that we teach them. It is simply too big a task.

Chapter 2 provides further insight into the experience of what happens to people when they go deaf – it details the personal consequences of hearing loss in individual lives. It too should not be taken for granted. Every person has a story to tell about their journey into deafness. Their story details the issues they need to address and resolve as part of the process of moving beyond deafness. It is the detail of each individual's story that provides the core working material for the rehabilitation programme. Chapter 3 provides the texture of what the journey out of deafness has been like for a number of people. For me, these stories were representative of the 58 people I interviewed during the course of my doctoral studies on living with hearing loss. What is most striking about these stories is that one works to move *beyond deafness* rather than seeking to get over it. Acceptance then is an odyssey in itself. Chapter 3 also highlights that rehabilitation is something that largely happens outside the clinic. Outside the clinic clients work to recreate their lives. One of the most critical things missing from current models of rehabilitation is the recognition that the clinic needs to work with the client beyond the bounds of speech perception tests and technological adjustments. Clinics need to engage with their clients as they seek to re-establish their lives, resolve family and personal difficulties, find useful employment and so on. The success of the rehabilitation programme outlined in Chapter 10 pivots on the fact that clinics will contract with their clients in a realistic way, to provide them with the support they need to achieve their life goals.

Chapter 4 is uniquely concerned with how clients actually get to clinics for assistance in the first place. It seeks to challenge the so-called myth of 'motivation'. Having appreciated the social conditioning which confronts Deafened people, it quickly becomes apparent that there are factors at work that readily predispose people to stay home and do nothing about their hearing loss. Further that there are many reasons clients or their families can find for not changing. Having recognized the marginality of our client group, active steps need to be taken to ensure that we work with our clients and their advocates to ensure that the many barriers to successful rehabilitation are overcome.

Psychosocial approaches to aural rehabilitation pivot on the assumption that you and your clients have engaged in a problem-solving process concerned with enabling them to overcome the difficulties which presently confront them. Chapters 5 and 6 are concerned with the attitudes, skills and approaches a practitioner requires in order to successfully deliver a client-centred, problem-solving intervention. Many existing aural rehabilitation programmes pivot around either the technology of interest or the perceptual tasks of immediate concern. Such interventions flow on logically from the many useful assessment techniques currently available. The client-centred approach sets these things aside for the present and seeks to address, in the group-process particularly, issues of immediate concern to the client. Assessment-centred therapy often means that the therapist 'asks the questions' and the answers can often be guessed in advance (by both client and practitioner). The client-centred, psychosocial approach is not so much concerned with asking questions as with facilitating a personal change process wherein the client learns to work through the social and emotional barriers that prevent them from communicating effectively. Chapter 5 examines various strategies for achieving this goal. Clearly, mastering the issues and techniques in Chapter 5 is critical to one being able to implement the psychosocial programme.

Chapter 6 examines a client-centred strategy for identifying and managing the various expectations everyone (including the practitioner) brings to the rehabilitation process. Practitioners often complain that their clients are not motivated or that they will not comply with the requirements of the rehabilitation process. Clients often have good reasons for such non-compliance and it is the responsibility of the practitioner to work with all people concerned with the rehabilitative outcome (client, partner, other practitioners) to identify competing and conflicting priorities that people might have and then work to resolve them. The Code-Müller Protocols provide a useful way to achieve these ends and to establish agreed priorities with clients within the framework of a rehabilitation plan. Being able to establish clear and agreed goals is critical to the successful implementation of the post-group phase of the rehabilitation programme.

Chapter 7 is concerned with how one delivers a programme concerned with psychosocial aspects of rehabilitation within the context of normal clinical life. It calls for a rethinking of current models of service delivery, by encouraging practitioners to think about how services might be best delivered from the clients' perspective, rather than simply seeking to calibrate our clients to fit into the logic and flow of diagnostic, assessment and/or surgical procedures.

Most Deafened people live on low incomes. In this new millennium, employment is critical to economic self-sufficiency and many clients look to the clinic to help in this regard. However, the provision of vocational services is often beyond the scope of most hearing clinics. In Chapter 8, practical, collaborative strategies for assisting clients seek out employment are examined.

Chapter 9 serves as a pause in the logical flow of this otherwise practical section of the book. Here the subtle nature of rehabilitation outcomes is examined from the clients' perspective. Notably, clients talk about how they have become reconnected to their world again, the sounds they like to hear, and how they have been able to resume their lives as they want to live them, as best they can under the circumstances. They do not talk about how well they did on a speech perception score. Rehabilitation is about re-establishing the ordinary. It is about facilitating people in the process of resuming their lives. Certainly in time, particularly as people access hearing services soon after the onset of deafness, we may look forward to people more readily retaining their employment and pre-deafness socio-economic position. In the meantime, it is reasonable to expect that the socio-economic position of Deafened people will gradually, but not dramatically, improve.

And finally we come to Chapter 10 – the psychosocial rehabilitation programme. This chapter, initially derived from the foundational work of Raymond Hetu and Louise Getty (1991), represents the overall focus of this text. Much has been changed and developed since the Montreal programme was developed in the late 1980s but I believe the materials presented in this chapter, and the conceptual and practical work which precedes it, are true to the spirit of the Montreal team. The programme was originally intended for newly industrially, Deafened people who had not begun to address their hearing difficulties. It was intended as a problem-solving process concerned with enabling Deafened people to address the difficulties hearing loss caused for them and their partners, to develop tactics and engage with technologies now available to them. But the programme works well for people who have also had exposure only to technology-based rehabilitation programmes and for people with differing degrees of hearing loss.

The programme pivots around three factors – recognizing the impact of hearing loss in one's life, understanding this impact, and developing the skills necessary to living more successfully with hearing loss. The programme is a workshop, not a course. It is intended to give participants the opportunity to develop the necessary attitudes, knowledge, skills and confidence in managing difficult communication settings in everyday life. It has been my experience that most clients know what to do in difficult communication settings, and this programme begins to enable them to turn knowledge into communicative competence. As one client, who had been to rehabilitation programmes for 20 years observed, while he had been to many services, this was the first time he had the opportunity to role-play and begin to master the various strategies he had been told so much about.

And so, while some of the materials in the programme may not be new to you, I trust that their application will be. Of course, the end is only the beginning. The conclusion of the intervention prepares both client and practitioner for the uncharted road ahead. These materials will change the way you work with your clients forever. I truly hope you enjoy using them.

Part I
Factors Impacting on the Psychosocial Predisposition of Clients with Hearing Loss

CHAPTER 1

A conceptual framework for a psychosocial approach to hearing rehabilitation

Introduction

People do not go deaf in a social vacuum. A variety of factors influence how people understand these things called 'disability' and 'deafness'. Attitudes and perceptions are important because they shape the way a community will respond to the needs of those affected. Some of the social factors impacting on Deafened people are:

- beliefs about a hearing world versus a deaf world;
- community attitudes to disability;
- professional practices;
- different technologies (hearing aids, cochlear implant, tactile aids, and various forms of sign language) and their respective applications.

All these factors shape the way people understand deafness, seek to manage and shape it and therein determine how Deafened people will associate with one another and the wider community. A belief in a deaf world and the positive aspects of disability provides the foundation for the Deaf community and the use of sign language. A belief in a hearing world and the positive aspects of hearing culture provides the foundation for the use of various technologies and hearing and speech. Of course, most people live in the Deaf World and the Hearing World. Irrespective of the level of hearing loss and the mode of communication used, when people with hearing loss get together they validate each others' experience of communication, the way they like to interact, sit, socialize and so on. The Deaf community has clearly described the cultural milieu in which signing Deaf people live. Indeed, the use of the capital 'D' is used as a mark of respect and recognition of the community, its language and ways of living. But Deafened adults (of all types and degrees of hearing loss, as well as the time in life when their hearing was lost) also have a shared cultural experience and social position. Much of this book will be taken up with describing it. It is equally important to recognize this cultural experience in a respectful manner. To this end, notions of Hearing Culture and the experience of being Deafened will be treated on an equal basis to that of the Deaf community.

Before thinking about how one might *help* Deafened people live out their lives (or how they might help themselves), it is important first of all to understand how our community has worked to shape attitudes to deafness, and therein sought to shape the behaviour and social position of Deafened people.

The philosopher Michel Foucault (1988) developed the idea of technologies of the self. Foucault thought that there were four interrelated factors that influenced how people would think of themselves (and be thought of by others) and seek to behave in everyday life. These formative factors are (see Figure 1.1):

- meaning and symbolism;
- institutions and professions;
- technologies and techniques;
- formation of the self.

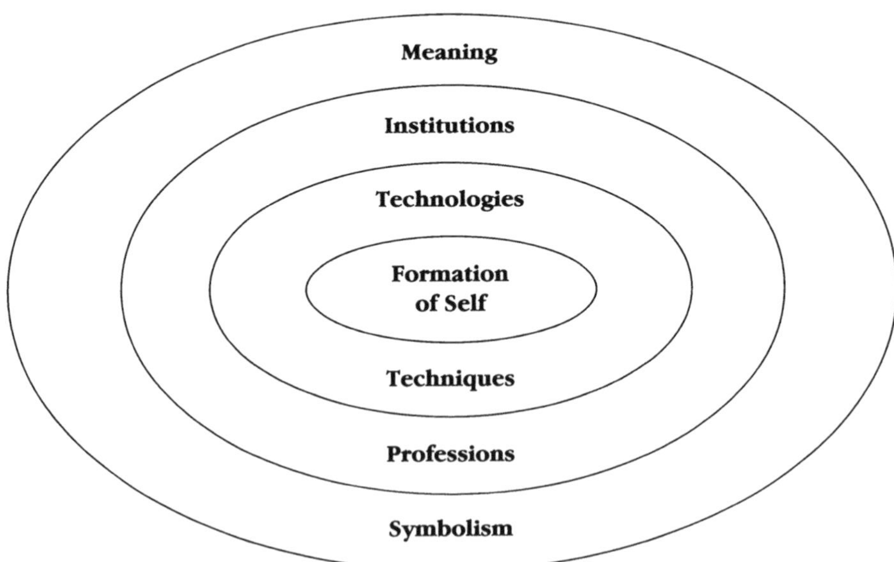

Figure 1.1: Technologies of the self.

At a social level, communities are actively engaged in addressing these factors through questions such as:

- what types of people do we see as ideal citizens?
- how do we produce such people?
- what skills, systems, procedures and technologies do we need to achieve this end?
- what institutional arrangements do we need to address these requirements?
- what changes in government policy or practice are indicated?
- what skills do our professionals require?
- what social networks need to be developed?

Of course, there are a variety of answers to questions such as these, with some being more popular, or at least more dominant, than others. Similarly, at the individual level, people ask such questions of themselves and seek to create themselves in ideal ways. Deafened people, for example, face a series of issues too, even if such issues are not apparent in their lives. These issues include questions such as:

- how am I to remake myself as a person who can communicate, so that I can live out my life as a social being, given the options (technologies, professions and funding) available to me?
- where will I go for help?
- what sort of person will I become?
- what will my life be like?

Later in the text we will examine personal stories and experiences of Deafened people as they seek to live out their lives, where the full meaning of these questions will become more apparent. But for now, let us simply focus on this question, of the need to remake oneself and all the meaning that it has within it. I use the notion of *remaking oneself* for this is what most Deafened people seek to do – they want to get back to being able to live their lives as they had been living it prior to deafness – or as near to it as they can get.

The first thing that strikes you is that there is a taken-for-granted assumption about the *normalness* of the life that the person has been living and that this is the life direction that they seek to re-establish – to get back on track as it were. This idea of normalness reflects assumptions about:

- the abnormalness of having a disability;
- the experience of disability disrupting a person's life in an undesirable way;
- the need to do *something* to get life *back on track*.

When people present at a hearing clinic for assistance they are not just seeking a hearing aid or a cochlear implant, they are seeking assistance to normalize their lives. It is important to stand back for a moment and think about the meanings and symbolism that support this notion of normality.

Meaning and symbolism

Normalization as a philosophy has shaped approaches to disability services since the early 1980s. The idea has been that an individual is a person first and has a disability second. This distinction between personhood and disability has been important. It has served to empower clients as people rather than being nothing more than a stereotyped idea of a disability or disease state. But like all concepts, it has been oversimplified. Certainly people do want to get on with their lives and be as much a part of society as they can be. However, several factors need to be taken into consideration here. Deafness is not simply a disability a person happens to have. As shall be demonstrated later in the text, deafness, and society's reaction to it, reaches into all aspects of people's lives and impacts on their life chances in education, employment, earning capacity, health and relationships. It is simply wrong to focus on disability as though there were no social consequences, as though one was *just* a person, who by the way, also just *happened* to be deaf. Life will not be normal for Deafened people until society changes; until they have an equal chance of getting a good job, earning a comparatively equal income and having relationships. Disability impacts on a person's life chances just as much as race and gender.

Just as many social practices have come to be understood as **sexist** and **racist** (that is, discriminatory on the basis of one's sex or race), many social practices are also ableist – that is they discriminate against a person on the basis of their disability (Davis, 1995). For Deafened people, the most common form of social ignorance is the assumption underlying **phonocentrism** (Corker, 1998) – that is, the assumption that all social interactions will be centred around speech and hearing, as though ideal communication could readily take place in a darkened, noisy room. Even with access to the best of technology, Deafened people will have trouble communicating in a noisy setting. Kaplan, Bailey and Garrestson's (1985) informative restaurant exercise highlights the fact that even a basic social function, such as going out for a meal, for Deafened people, is an experience where they confront the limits of technology, and society's awareness of the needs of Deafened people. Indeed, do not many so-called hearing people have trouble communicating in restaurants and cafés these days? It is evident that the present design of communicative social interactions do not work well – not just for Deafened people, but for many people generally. So the ideal of seeking to become normal, as in this example, is a silly one. Why is it that we think we are having a good time when we sit in a noisy café and yell at each other all night and go home with a sore throat, having really not understood much of what was said by most people all night? These social settings need to be changed so that they *accommodate* everyone's need for access to communication, not just Deafened people.

The point here is that the search for normality may at times be a misguided one and that the idea of normality can actually be oppressive to people. Where oppression or discrimination exists, we seek not to reform the individual who is oppressed, but to change the social foundations of oppression, in this instance by designing social settings that use soft furnishings and better layout, where the underside of dining tables are lined with sound-absorbing materials, coupled with promoting styles of interaction that make it easier for people to hear. This is not as bizarre as it seems. Fifteen years ago who would have thought that you could go out to a smoke-free restaurant or that communities would promote the health hazards related to alcohol consumption? Change can occur, it just takes time and effort.

In addition to notions of normality, there are four other meaning systems we need to think about. These are:

- medical versus social model of disability;
- dependency versus independence;
- overcoming versus living with disability;
- hearing versus disability culture.

Medical versus social model of disability

The **bio-mechanical model** of the body has been developed over several centuries and has stemmed from pathology-based medicine that located disease processes within certain deficient organs or body systems (see Foucault, 1991d). The logic follows that disease, illness and/or disability could be managed by simply identifying and repairing or replacing the deficient organ. The bio-mechanical model of the body also became associated with the **tragedy model** of disability (Finkelstein, 1980). The tragedy model depicted the onset of disability as literally a terrible thing that had happened to a person. It was a state to be avoided and where possible, overcome or eliminated. For as will be seen below, disability, certainly in previous centuries, had a devastating impact on one's life chances.

The **social model of disability** (Finkelstein 1980; Oliver, 1993b) understands disability as a normal part of everyday life, not something to be overcome, but to be integrated into the flow of everyday activities. Indeed, as David Pfeiffer observes, it is only a matter of time until everyone experiences some form of disability first hand. The difficulty identified under the social model of disability is that society has structured itself around assumptions of able-bodiment – as though everyone can hear in dark and noisy restaurants. However, with some 22 per cent (Wilson et al., 1999) of the community experiencing impaired hearing, such assumptions are clearly ill-founded. For even if each hearing-impaired person tried to speak with only one other non-hearing-impaired person (such as a partner) in a social setting each week, then half of the population would regularly experience communication problems.

While the medical model seeks to *fix up* breakdowns in the body, the social model seeks to rectify breakdowns in social arrangements. Certainly both models of the body have something to offer the Deafened person, particularly if the patronizing notions of the tragedy model (i.e. you poor thing) are dispensed with.

Dependency versus independence

The nineteenth century was a time of massive social upheaval in Europe and America. Many people were displaced by social revolution, war and the process of social change that resulted from urbanization and industrialization. Societies became particularly concerned about managing the poorer classes, particularly out of a fear to prevent further social unrest. People with disabilities were one group that became the focus of attention from social administrators. Administrators were concerned with the care and management of people unable to provide for themselves. Throughout the century, community values began to promote the idea that people should be economically self-sufficient; that they could provide for themselves. At the same time, parish-based systems of welfare (alms giving) began to diminish. Without access to employment (land-based or urban) or welfare, people were literally destitute and on the streets. As part of their efforts to control this mass of people, and to separate out those who deserved help (i.e. people with disabilities) from those who did not (e.g. people who might now be referred to as benefit-scroungers or long-term unemployed and/or people without employable skills – those deemed not wanting to work), administrators set up workhouses and systems that sought to institutionalize disabled people for the purposes of preparing them for work. Unfortunately few people actually graduated from their asylums as those most able to work were needed to maintain the institution as an economically viable unit (Pfeiffer, 1994; Hogan, 1997).

As part of the community's push to ensure that people provided for themselves, steps were taken to ensure that these poorhouses were less than comfortable (Dean, 1992). The social push for creating a society based on personal self-sufficiency, coupled with the negativity associated with being dependent on an institution for social support, meant that citizens began to see dependency on others as an undesirable state. Ideally, one would seek to look after oneself and therein be independent.

These days, being independent means very specific things to disabled people, not least of which has been getting out of those institutions that were developed in the last century. But it also means being able to carry on life as one wants to live it, to have control over personal decision-making, to be physically autonomous, to choose one's social relations and to be able to engage in activities without relying on others. No one would dispute these ideals as things to be sought after and promoted. However, proponents of the social model argue that the idea of independence has been taken too far and has only been focused on disabled people while ignoring the fact that we are all dependent on each other to a certain extent, it is simply that we take for granted many of these social dependencies as they are designed to suit a society centred on able-bodiedness. The threat of the millennium bug highlighted the point. As the millennium approached, the dependency of whole communities on socially provided systems such as water, gas, electricity, banks, supermarkets, roads, traffic lights, public transport systems and computers became quite apparent.

The social model of disability does not promote the idea of maintaining disabled people as dependent. Rather, it seeks to highlight the fact that the modern community is an interdependent one and that there are many assumptions about able-bodiment that underpin it. Rather than making disabled people fit into these arrangements, they simply ask that we recognize the extent to which society supports each of us in our activities of daily living and to ensure that such processes are accessible to all. Such accommodations have been made to the physical environment (e.g. ramps and rails) but not to the communication environment.

Overcoming versus living with a disability

In everyday magazines that one can buy at the supermarket one can readily find stories about some individual with a disability who has overcome the limitations of their condition to some degree. The deaf musician, the crippled rock climber, and so on. These magazines idealize *great* disabled people as those who can live as though they did not have a disability. However, ideal disabled people are not pretend able-bodied people, they are who they are. Getting on with life is not about denying one's disability, but living as a citizen with equal rights and social responsibilities, irrespective of how these roles come to be expressed. It follows that the goal of hearing rehabilitation is not to enable Deafened people to hear in a darkened, noisy room, but to enable them to access communication environments through technologies, hearing strategies and social change.

Hearing culture versus deaf culture

Most Deafened people belong to the hearing world. They were born into it, grew up in it and have all their networks established within it. As part of their rehabilitative experience, most will seek to maintain their place within the hearing world. However, as noted already, it would be wrong to deny the many positive things that deafness brings into people's lives, even if those positives are yet to be apparent to the client (for instance their partner's snoring does not bother them).

It should now be apparent that a whole range of factors influence how individuals and communities see disability. Where disability is concerned, western society is currently in a state of social transition. On the one hand the rights of disabled people are being recognized more and more (see, for example, disability rights laws) while, on the other hand, disability is seen as something to be truly avoided. Expectant parents seek to avoid having a disabled child while processes of euthanasia are openly discussed as a solution to physical dependency. Community attitudes are still very much caught up in the medico-tragedy model of disability and reflect on disability as a negative state of dependency to be avoided wherever possible.

When Deafened people present for rehabilitation, they are very much aware of these competing value systems and what it means for them to be disabled or to be labelled as such. Most specifically, because they are unable to participate readily in conversation and speech, they routinely disrupt the everyday flow of social interactions. Being perceived as unable to partake in even the most basic forms of taken-for-granted living, people perceive the disabled person as socially incompetent (Giddens, 1991; Noble, 1991). Giddens (1991) points out that the essential criterion for agency is competence: 'routine control of the body is integral to the very nature both of agency and of being accepted by others as competent' (p. 56). Put plainly, people think Deafened adults are stupid. While most Deafened people would like to see the end of such discrimination at the social level, they seek out help in the first instance simply to avoid or minimize the extent to which communities might notice that they cannot hear.

According to Giddens, the opposite of shame and its associated fear is self-esteem and 'confidence in the integrity and value of the narrative of self-identity' (p. 66) – something referred to in the Deaf Community as Deaf Pride. Giddens (1991) and Goffman (1973) hold that the very promise or threat of a social encounter poses a crises of individual identity because the person is confronted with a struggle between cultural pride or personalized shame. Identity then is a social phenomenon, a product of social engagement. Becoming deafened disrupts the narrative of personal identity. Deafened people cannot control the interactive processes in the same way as hearing people because hearing people's rules for communication are privileged over those of Deafened people and because Deafened people lack the necessary social organization and power to contest this relationship. Feelings of guilt and shame related to the experience of having this disability reflect the internalization of a social problem as a personal ill (Mills, 1970). Such feelings reflect an unresolved dissonance within the individual because daily living cannot be reconciled with the meanings and expected behaviours legitimated by the ableist discourse (Jung, 1983). Individuals present at clinics seeking assistance for the dilemmas they confront in daily living. However, many of the required solutions are inaccessible to clients because hearing therapies do not take into account adequately the very psychosocial dramas that hearing tactics create.

Institutions and professions and their technologies and techniques

Just as people do not go deaf in a social vacuum, nor do they remake themselves as Deafened people in social isolation. Institutions were developed in the nineteenth century to address disability issues of the day, so today governments and communities have set up processes to address this *problem* known as deafness. The options one has with regard to rehabilitation are determined by the social factors already noted. Specifically, rehabilitation options are determined by:

- the community's attitude towards disability (e.g. the medical social continuum);
- the thinking of the day;
- support offered by government and private funding processes;
- the skills and technologies presently available for assistance;
- models of intervention (public versus private; self-help versus professional).

Depending on how a system tries to remake Deafened people and into what it tries to change them, it will draw upon a range of technologies and rehabilitative techniques. Technologies include both communication instruments (hearing aids, cochlear implants, assistive listening devices) as well as diagnostic and surgical tools (oto-acoustic emissions, brain-stem evoked responses, electrode insertion tools and so on). Techniques include strategies for teaching people to communicate either orally (e.g. speech discrimination exercises, social tactics) or in sign language and might also encompass assertiveness training and confidence building techniques. Rehabilitation services generally seek to produce Deafened people as those who live in the hearing world, while not taking into account adequately the extent to which they are and will remain Deafened people. This text seeks to remedy this limitation of existing rehabilitation programmes.

Formation of the self

For most people, deafness is acquired in adult life. However, for those who acquire quite severe to profound loss of hearing, their impairment may have begun to onset quite early in life and in turn have progressively fallen away in later adult life. Prior to hearing loss, most Deafened people had a perception of themselves as *normal*. As we shall see later in the text, we take our *identity* from what we can do and with whom we do things. People, for example, may define themselves by their employment, where they live, the activities they like to do and the people with whom they share their lives. Deafness shapes identity in a special way for it determines the extent to which one can participate in many relationships while pre-empting, in many cases, how one will be treated within those relationships. Prior to hearing loss, people had a commonsense way of doing things and saw themselves, perhaps not at a conscious level, as living out their lives in some notion of able-bodied bliss. The onset of deafness disrupts this vision and challenges one's very notion of who you are, how you fit into the world and how you will live out the rest of your life. The onset of deafness signals not just the loss of hearing, but also the loss of a sense of self and often the subsequent loss of employment and possibly of a life partner. For those who acquire lesser degrees of hearing loss, it may not be so much the loss of employment that is the problem but the loss of promotional opportunities; not the loss of a life partner but the loss of an active social life. When individuals present for rehabilitation they clearly want more than just their hearing back and it would be naïve of the practitioner to think that a piece of technology is going to undo all that has happened to date.

Deafened people engage in the rehabilitative process in the hope of making some sense of what has happened to them and to develop a strategy (consisting of technologies, skills, behaviours and attitudes) to get their lives back on track. The view they had of themselves is now gone (or within the rehabilitation process they will come to realize this loss of self at a conscious level). There is a rupture between who one thinks one is and the things one could do and the person one is now and the things one can now (not) do. Specifically, daily life is now problematic in a way that it never was before and the problem pervades every aspect of life, or so it seems. This is because hearingness (or phonocentricism) is a fact of life at the beginning of the twenty-first century. As the sociologist Emile Durkheim noted, anyone who breaches the taken-for-grantedness of a social fact gets punished. A *social fact*, Durkheim noted, can 'be recognised by the power of external coercion which it exercises or is capable of exercising over individuals, and the presence of this power may be recognised in its turn either by the resistance offered every individual who tends to violate it' (1971: 63).

A joke I heard on the radio recently illustrates the point. A woman rings up her bank and asks to speak with the bank manager. The officer answering the call is apologetic, informing the woman that she cannot speak to the manager as the person died the evening before.

'Fine,' says the woman and hangs up. Some ten minutes later she rings back and the same person answered the telephone:

> 'May I speak with the bank manager please?' she asks.
> 'I'm sorry,' replies the bank officer, 'the manager died last night. You'll have to ring back when we have a new manager.'
> 'OK,' says the woman and hangs up. A little while later she rings back again.
> 'May I speak with the bank manager please?' she asks.
> 'Are you deaf or something,' replies the bank officer. 'I told you, the bank manager died last night!'
> 'I know,' says the caller. 'I just enjoy hearing the news!'

Now despite modern society's dislike of the banking sector, the point of this story is that to ask for things to be repeated, as though one were deaf, attracts anger, insult and correction; one is put down and identified as incompetent based on the assumption that one cannot hear, for simply breaching the social assumption (fact) about how everyday communication should occur – that one person will say something and that the other will immediately respond. The fact of the matter is that our everyday sense of security stems from the extent to which most of our activities of daily living can be taken for granted. Indeed, do not all these New Age self-help books on stress talk about getting things under control and that stress stems from uncertainty in this so-called age of rapid change?

A person's sense of well-being stems from the predictability of everyday life (Giddens, 1991). Daily rituals promote a sense of security. As some people say, 'I just can't start the day without a cup of coffee (tea, etc.)'. It follows then that the absence of predictability results in fear and anxiety for some and annoyance for others. Deafened people may well go into banks filled with fear and anxiety about how they will fare with oral communication through bullet-proof glass while planning to manage the patronizing anger and insults of an ignorant and intolerant teller. As Goffman (1973) put it, the avoidance of being put down is very much about being able to manage the presentation of oneself as competent in everyday social settings. Yet for the Deafened person this is all but impossible as deafness prevents them from playing by phonocentric rules. They are left with the options of trying to participate in conversations knowing that at any time they may be perceived as socially incompetent, while trying to manage breakdowns effectively and in a discreet fashion. But it does not have to be this way. Participating in conversations, particularly in difficult settings, might be likened to slowly walking across hot coals while maintaining a serene smile! OK for some but hell for most! And as the research shows, managing such situations (lack of control with no useful coping strategies) is the most damaging form of all stress (Carlson and Hatfield, 1992).

When the rules for everyday living no longer work, Durkheim reminds us that people find themselves in a state of normlessness, what he referred to as *anomie* (see Figure 1.2). In addition to normlessness, anomie can be thought of as having an enduring sense of social uncertainty and hence fear, coupled with a hypersensitivity to difficult situations (like banks), a tendency to withdraw socially (as though one gradually cuts off all difficult social ties and is shrinking away like a bonsai plant – hence the notion of the bonsai effect) and one experiences an enduring sense of a shock or

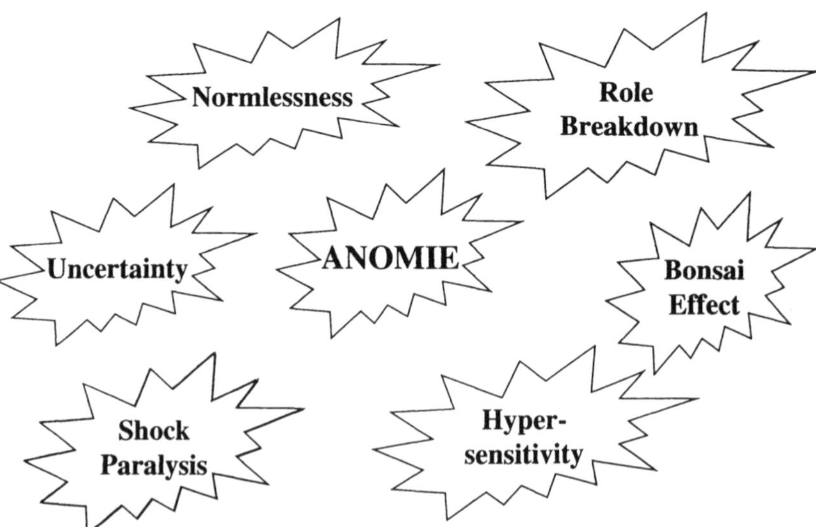

Figure 1.2: Anomie.

paralysis response (Spencer, 2000), that is typified by having a sense of frozen-numbness in situations where one just does not know what to do next. For most Deafened people, anomie is experienced within intense moments of communication breakdown in everyday settings. It is not a complete experience of anomie – one can go home and, within the confines of domestic safety, life has a certain predictability; things can be controlled. Yet, when confronted with a group situation, being unable to respond appropriately, feeling confused, fearful, socially stuck, disconnected from the mainstream of society and unsure of what to do, the decision to withdraw into social isolation looks to be a good option. Many Deafened people do in fact withdraw from society as much as they can because life has suddenly become quite unpredictable and this loss of predictability is coupled with a loss of self-confidence and a blurring of identity (Giddens, 1991).

No longer being sure how to behave reduces one's self-confidence. One's sense of identity is in turn destablized since the sense of self often exists in the context of who one is in relation to others and idealized notions of who one is or ought to be (Jung, 1983). Identity then is very much a verb. A person is someone who does certain things, with certain groups of people in particular settings. When individuals are no longer able to fulfil these roles, their place in such interactions is threatened. One becomes less sure of everything. As Jung remarked, once fear has taken hold, and avoidance behaviours set in, one engages in a negative and downward spiral that can only ever really be overcome by confronting the fears themselves:

> The moment of an outbreak of neurosis is not just a matter of chance; as a rule it is most critical. It is usually the ***moment when a new psychological adjustment, that is, a new adaptation, is demanded*** (Jung, 1983: 49, emphasis in the original).

The presence of stress, then, is an indicator that the individual needs to learn new ways to behave. Anomie indicates the need for change. The anomic experience is a moment wherein the individual experiences fear as a primal emotion (it is literally a shocking experience) that is associated with a whole range of reactions within the sympathetic nervous system (sweating, blood pressure, pulse rate, digestive or sleep problems). The emotional and physiological responses are coupled with cognitive shifts in the way individuals perceive certain stimuli and themselves in relation to it. Clearly, the fight/flight response is activated. However, for most it does not stay activated at the conscious level very long. Rather, the brain creates a shortcut (called a ***heuristic*** (Baron and Byrne, 1987)) for coping with the perceived threat to the self. The intensity of being confronted with being a non-person becomes displaced into a stress and/or avoidance reaction. Reactive behaviours result and are charged emotionally as a conditioned response.

The key emotions often associated with deafness, such as having a sense of embarrassment, the need to fit in and denial, are in fact tertiary experiences. The secondary level is a sense of shame and inferiority and the primal level, as already noted, is fear. Most particularly, it is a fear of rejection and the complete loss of self – the experience of being completely engulfed by the seething sea of emotion that underpins the flight/fight scenario as it plays out before you, or at least in the imagination. Giddens (1991) argues that anxiety is substitutive – that is, rather than containing all these things in conscious awareness, our minds shrink all these emotions down into the idea that 'I just don't like going some places.' The very threat of having to go to such places brings out an anxiety response in the form of compliance (putting up with difficult situations by pretending that everything is OK), conflict (when things break down or as one attempts, either unsuccessfully or as the result of arguments, to avoid social engagement) or self-isolation (avoidance behaviours) that serve to mask all the underlying issues noted above. As Karen Horney (1959: 314) observes, these behaviours are the three faces of basic anxiety (moving toward people, against them or away from them):

> The dominant attitude, however, is the one that most strongly determines actual conduct. It represents those ways and means of coping with others in which the particular person feels most at home. Thus a detached person will as a matter of course use all the unconscious techniques for keeping others at a safe distance because he feels at a loss in any situation that requires close association with them. Moreover, the ascendant attitude is often but not always the one most acceptable to the person's conscious mind (Horney, 1959: 314).

And so a picture begins to emerge of the parameters that potentially underpin the psychological state of the Deafened person who feels under threat (though not every one feels under threat or under threat to the same extent). Confronted with the inability to carry out everyday interactions, the individual experiences, to differing degrees, fear, guilt, anxiety, worry, sadness, grief, anger, frustration and a loss of intimacy. Certainly the description here of the stressed Deafened person is a stereotype – not everyone experiences all these things all the time, or even ever. Indeed, as David Wilson's (1997) work has demonstrated, evidence at a population level suggests an absence of psycho-pathology among Deafened people generally.

These then are aspects of the psychological experience of coming to live with deafness as described by Deafened people and as I have been able to bring them together into some sort of coherent story based on the literature. Even despite this stereotyping, the experience of anomie (be it mild or severe) has symptoms of fear; it contains the threat of exposure of being seen as stupid and a consequent sense of social inadequacy. It has an experience of the soul, as it were, being laid bare in a public space (they think I am stupid, but I'm only deaf) and its accompanying feelings of shame and rejection. This is the journey into a loss of the sense of self and it is a journey that each Deafened person experiences even if not to the same degree (see Figures 1.3 and 1.4). With each new client what is interesting is to establish the extent to which fear-based behaviours are present, and to what extent the individual is aware of these, for this is where the journey back into personhood begins.

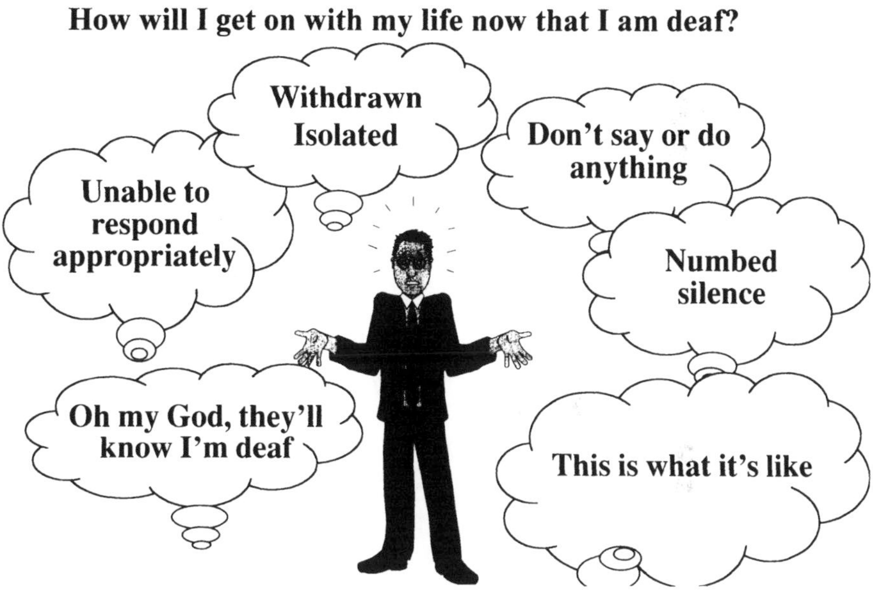

Figure 1.3: Deafness dilemma.

Identity and a sense of pride

One's sense of identity is dependent on what one does, and with whom one does it. It can be seen then that one's sense of identity is a dynamic thing, it changes as life changes and has different aspects depending on what one is doing. The key issue for Deafened people following the onset of deafness is maintaining an ongoing narrative of the self – having a story about themselves that connects the past with the present, while creating a future. Deafened people have a will to get on with life, to create

Trust –
I can't rely on myself
Can't function –
ashamed about it
Unable to
respond
appropriately –
feel inferior
Fear
Who am I really?
Isolation

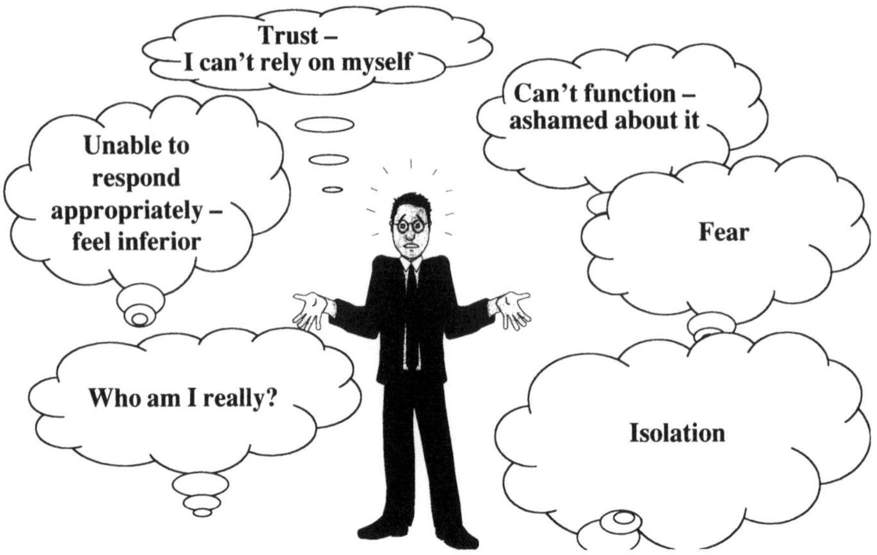

Figure 1.4: Key issues of the self.

themselves anew. It is the role of rehabilitation to facilitate this *will to be*. If the road into the loss of self centres around role breakdown, *identity-based dissonance* and an associated sense of shame (see Figure 1.5), then the road back into selfhood pivots on evolving a new and valued sense of self that transforms that sense of shame into an enduring experience of personal pride and satisfaction with life. Pride here can be defined as being made up of:

- self-confidence;
- ability;
- self-esteem;
- security;
- a sense of the future;
- a sense of where I fit in the world.

The re-establishment of selfhood (see Figure 1.6) is achieved by reversing the processes set up by the dynamics of shame and marginalization. Confronted with an experience of anomie, it is recalled that Deafened people experience a sense of loss of self, and of the capacity to participate socially, in an adequate fashion. Before a sense of self-worth can be established, the rehabilitation process seeks first to acknowledge what has

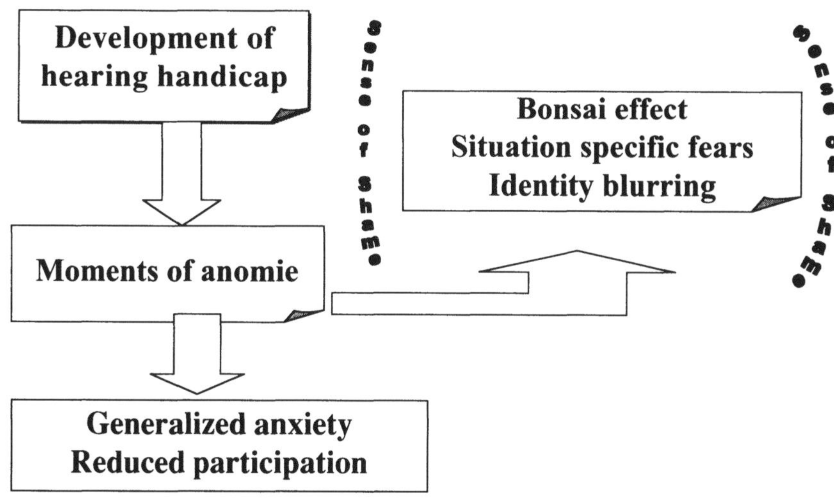

Figure 1.5: Path into the loss of the real self.

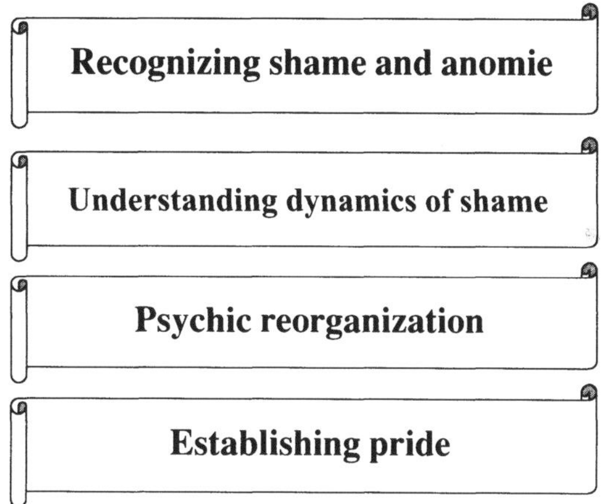

Figure 1.6: The path into selfhood.

already taken place in the life of the Deafened person, to recognize the dynamics of shame as they have occurred in people's everyday lives and to come to see the consequences the anomic experience has had on self-esteem – that one feels embarrassed, or has a sense of self-shame that may manifest itself in symptoms of stress.

Critical to the process of reclaiming the self is enabling Deafened people to recognize:

- the way they have been depicted socially;
- the words people have used with regards to deafness, the stereotypes others hold;
- the things societies have sought to do to Deafened people in order to make them fit in;
- the extent to which one's sense of self has been constructed in conformity with the medico-tragedy model of disability;
- the pressures placed on people around the notion of dependency;
- the meaning of anxiety and stress-based responses in their lives;
- the extent to which they too may have been denied an education, a financial living, a love-filled life, and a social network, not because their character was somehow inherently flawed, but because of the way our community has chosen to respond to deafness.

This process is not about opening up a psychological Pandora's box (although for some, a level of counselling may be beneficial) – but a process of sorting out the self (see Figure 1.7) through legitimating the shared experience of being a part of a minority group within a larger society. It is about laying the groundwork for the reorganization of one's sense of personhood; about learning to see oneself differently while discharging a lot of emotional baggage collected during various engagements with

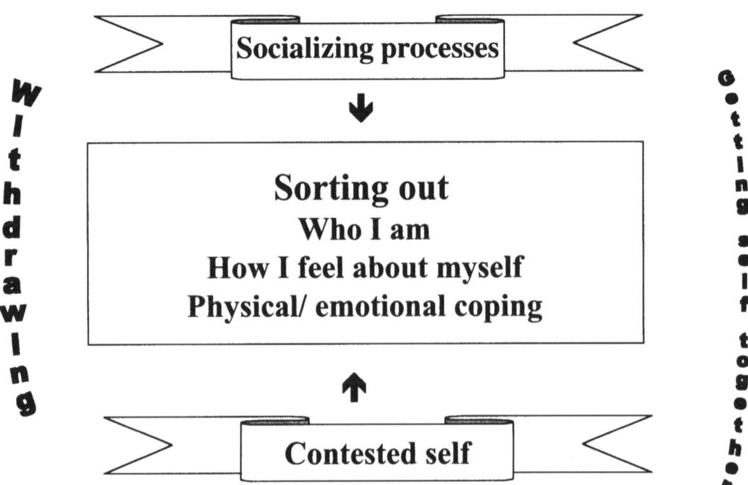

Figure 1.7: The social self.

phonocentricism. Pride, or a sense of self-worth then emerges as the validity of the self becomes apparent – *it's not my fault; there's a reason for all of this*; suddenly it all makes sense and a sense of wholeness begins to emerge. One can stand and face the world as a Deafened person and feel strong. This emergent sense of strength (for it happens as a process, not overnight) can be seen in the way one begins to act. One feels gradually more:

- confident
- sure
- OK
- connected
- goal-oriented.

The formation of the self can then be understood as concurrent, working through of a series of psychological challenges that Erik Erickson (1965) first attributed to people across the life span (see Figure 1.8). But these are not stages but states of being; continua that one moves along or between throughout the rest of one's life as a Deafened person. In Figure 1.8 I have tried to depict the process of identity change confronting the Deafened person, based upon Erickson's foundational work. Within the first four levels one addresses the issues of identity formation and personal survival while the remaining three are concerned with the integration of identity and self-actualization. Linked into these identity states are a series of emotional responses and physiological states (Figure 1.9). The emergence

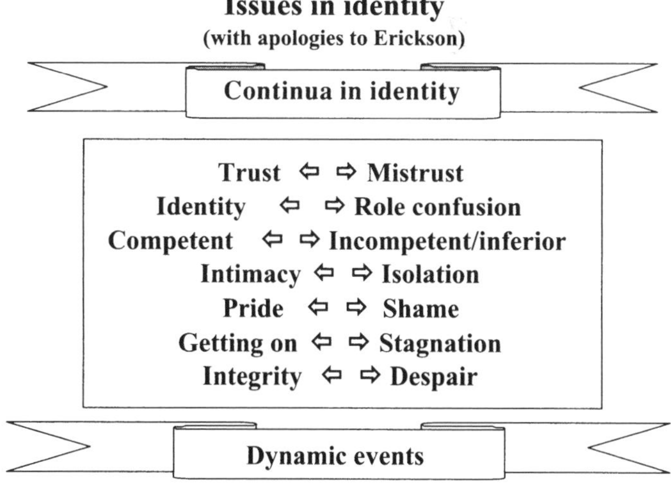

Figure 1.8: Social psychology of acquired hearing loss.

of the sense of self (as either coherent or threatened) occurs as a result of these three interrelated processes (self-awareness, emotion (the *charging* process as it were) and the physical)) and the configurations of alignments that result.

The initial issues concerning the individual then centre on the extent to which social life becomes predictable or trustworthy, that individuals can know what will happen in social interactions and be happy with these outcomes; that they can be clear about who they are and the roles to be played out; that they can feel competent to interact with a sense of worth and that they can be a part of things. Then, as people who are happy with their lot in life, they can confidently go about their business, moving on with the goals they have established for their life with a sense of wholeness and well-being.

The idea of these things being a continuum becomes apparent in daily living. Nothing is perfect. No one feels wholly together all or even most of the time. Rather, one moves along the slide between the ideal and negative state so that one's emotional alignment looks a lot like the knobs on a graphic equalizer, with each person finding the arrangement of emotional states that becomes his or her ongoing life, while allowing for the impact of day-to-day events.

All these factors pivot around two key themes that we will examine constantly in this text and in therapy. These are *coherency* and *continuity*

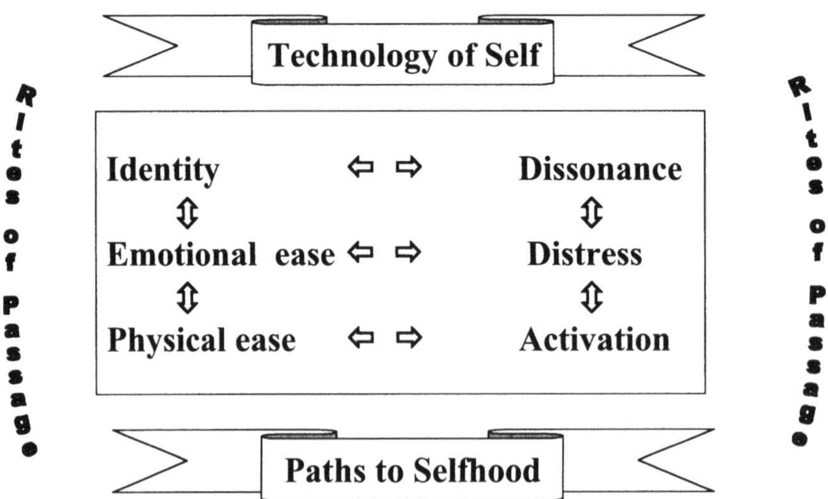

Figure 1.9: Maintaining a wholesome self.

(Moore, 1994). How do clients make sense of what has happened to them in their lives and can they see a way forward?

It is the purpose of the rehabilitative experience, be it engaged spontaneously through life or through the facilitation offered by a clinic or service, to enable the individual to make the transition from the anomic state, back into a sense of self. It is the purpose of this book to help facilitate this journey. In this context then, rehabilitation is not simply about the application of technologies or communication therapies. It is about enabling clients to:

- recognize where their lives are;
- engage in a problem-solving process;
- start to make changes across a variety of life domains (identity, emotion, body);
- remake themselves into something in which they find meaning and peace.

In my earlier work (Hogan, 1996) I described the journey into deafness as a cochlear odyssey. People shared a common point of departure, the onset of hearing loss, but were left with few clues as to where their lives would go or the level of benefit they could expect to obtain. Rehabilitation is about working with the Deafened adult to define the purpose of the journey, the itinerary as it were, the experiences to be gained and the outcomes to be achieved. We strive to do more than just give people an experience of sound, but to enable Deafened people to get on with their lives in a positive way.

CHAPTER 2

The onset of deafness

Introduction

In Chapter 1 we examined, in a theoretical way, the issues confronting Deafened adults. In this and the following chapter we examine the issues from the perspective of Deafened people themselves.

There is a community adage that states that *if you don't know where you're going, you'll end up somewhere else*. This statement is particularly true for people who go deaf and find themselves engaged in hearing services. Deafened adults and providers of hearing services spontaneously engage in a process concerned to *remake* the deafened adult back into a hearing person – or as near as they can get to this goal. Yet this apparently simple task can get awfully complicated, partly because both service users and service providers lack clarity about the exact nature of the task at hand. Certainly the issues about the specific applications of hearing aids and cochlear implants may be clear to many, but what may not be so clear are the broader psychosocial aspects of the rehabilitation process. What are they? Do they impact on the rehabilitation process and if so, to what extent?

If rehabilitation can loosely be termed a process concerned with enabling clients to relearn to live as they once were, or as near to it as possible, then we really must understand what has been lost and what the nature of the quest at hand is really all about. The process of hearing rehabilitation is about enabling clients to make sense of and to get on with their lives, in the same way as before their impairment, but doing so in a very different fashion – it's about doing the same things differently; it's about being the same person but in a different way; it's about carving out a decent future from a troubled and often traumatic past (Hogan, 1998b).

This chapter commences with a recounting of the experiences of people who have lost their hearing. It then proceeds to explain in psychosocial terms, how rehabilitation is constituted as a process concerned with the remaking of one's self.

Onset

Onset refers to the experience of acquiring profound hearing loss. It examines the experience of the onset and consequences of acquired severe to profound hearing loss from the analytical perspective offered by a sociology informed by post-structuralism and post-modernism. One seeks not just to gain an understanding of what happens to people following the onset of deafness, but also to analyse the processes that create and sustain such outcomes. In particular, what is it about the experience of acquired hearing loss, particularly profound hearing loss, that leads some people to pursue one type of self-formation over another? Is the experience of being deafened merely audiological, or is it shaped by social relations? In turn, what services does the community offer Deafened people and on what basis? To what outcomes do social interventions lead Deafened people?

This examination of onset is structured by the differing experiences encountered by people as a result of the *timing of, consequences arising from, and the extent of the onset* of acquired hearing loss. People may go deaf at any age. The timing of onset can have a direct bearing on the type of language skills they may develop, the education they may receive and the type of employment opportunities available which they may access. Such consequences are examined in relation to respondents' personal and social networks, family, friends, school and work. Through their experiences, Deafened people engage discourses that configure onset as a personal rather than social process and that privilege the voice of science over their own.

The maintenance of personal networks is challenged by hearing loss. The extent of disruption resulting from loss is constituted by the extent to which one is able to continue relationships and/or maintain a proximity to one's previous lifestyle. If continuity can be achieved, things can appear as business as usual. Support is there and remains. Life goes on. It is just a setback as in the game Snakes and Ladders; only the stakes are higher. Given the way the game is played, lost ground can be recovered even if extra effort is entailed. Following onset, the rules of participation in the game change. The question becomes not whether one is likely to win the game, but on what basis, if at all, one may be allowed to play.

For some people, despite the extent of loss, disruption can be minimized. They can get on with life without making substantive adjustments because they have gained or retained sufficient communication skills, supportive social networks or (even minimally) aidable thresholds.

Following onset, some ability to hear may remain. Depending on the point at which this hearing ability cuts in, it may be possible to enhance the strength and range of sounds being sent to the inner ear through the use of conventional hearing aids – hence the term ***aidable thresholds***. Those who cannot avoid disruption and cannot continue as before, or as near before, are the worst affected.

With the onset of deafness, the person, as he or she has been known by others, is gone. Rapid onset plunges a person into a completely different world, while slow onset can be likened to a slow migration. The experience of coming to live with acquired hearing loss must therefore be understood as one of a range of possible practices shaped by 'contexts, material and symbolic, physical and emotional, social and psychic' (Dowsett, 1994: 71). One is different yet one stays the same. Communication is now different but the rules for social engagement stay the same. The consequences of onset are determined by the social, by the manner in which one's networks cope and adjust as everyone learns to live in a different manner.

Neither the personal nor the social consequences of acquired hearing loss are necessarily equivalent to the extent of impairment sustained (Lutman, Brown and Coles, 1987; Noble, 1991). The physiological loss of a small amount of hearing for a teacher may be of greater personal and social consequence for that person than a large amount of physiological loss sustained by a blue-collar worker who lives alone. The net effect of acquired hearing loss must therefore be evaluated in the light of the specific consequences that arise for the Deafened person, such as rejection by those in one's immediate network or becoming unemployed. For the most part the discussion will focus on people who acquire severe to profound hearing loss. However, clinical experience has shown that people with varying degrees of deafness do indeed have much in common.

Early onset: family, friends and school

When a person is deafened as a minor, families experience a crisis. Parents choose a communication system for their child, a strategy wherein the impairment can be incorporated as far as possible into the everyday, common-sense practice of family living – business (almost) as usual. Such decision-making is not a straightforward process and is influenced by shifting educational philosophies. Jean is a young person who was deafened at an early age and who now has a cochlear implant. Her experience highlights problems inherent in the system.

The family was confronted with a series of decisions, the most serious of which was where to continue the child's education and in what mode.

At that time children went away to boarding school where they learnt to communicate in sign language. This option proved unacceptable to the family as they regarded this mode as abnormal and the placement of the child in boarding school an infringement of their sense of identity as a family. By definition, the mode of education reflected a conceptualization of normality, which, on reflection, the family rejected. In turn, to achieve the family's goal, Jean's mother engaged in a process of self-advocacy, wherein she sought the outcomes she desired for her child and her family. In dealing with 'helpers', Jean's parents expressed anger and resentment over the power they exerted in their lives as different perspectives came into conflict. The family presented as having engaged in a crisis and as having had to learn to cope with forceful technocrats. The professionals they initially engaged were unhelpful to the point of conflict. In coming to terms with their position, the parents defined their own strategy and pursued it. In so doing, they enlisted allies, such as teachers who agreed with them, to substantiate their position. They maintained their sense of identity as a family and in so doing articulated a sense of 'normal for us'.

Jean completed school in a type of mainstreamed social isolation. For the parents, coherence and continuity were constituted by Jean being seen to do the same things as other young people, going to the same school and playing the same games. However, Jean recalls the experience:

> I didn't have too many friends back then. I had enough to well ... I didn't talk to anyone really ... and there was classes ... I didn't like it being there not being able to understand anything, having to wait for someone to tell me what was going on. I think maybe I was quite depressed.

Throughout her narrative, Jean's mother maintains a sense of the tragedy of deafness. The consequences of deafness are shared by close relatives or surviving friends and, as such, it is not necessarily the Deafened person who has the problem.

Jan, another person deafened while at school, points out that onset constitutes a double crisis for young people who have to cope with their loss of hearing as well as their families grief:

> The sad thing is that my parents couldn't cope with what happened and anytime that I wanted to talk about it I was rebuffed and the subject was changed immediately.

In a reverse scenario, Jan's family goes along with the philosophy of the day, which in her case was one of lip-reading and speech. Practice continues to shape association and identity. Jan's family did not have to countenance systemic change within the household whereas Jean's did.

The point is focused in a third family who lived in a culture where living with an impairment was especially marginal. In Maria's country of origin, deafness was culturally viewed as a taboo, a sign of bad luck or indicative of the sins of the family. Maria went deaf at a young age and was not allowed to return to school. The family bribed the school to take her back. Within her culture, the onset of an impairment signalled the end of Maria's utility – the education system offered no form of intervention. There was no system of hearing rehabilitation, so Maria taught herself to lip-read. Upon her return to school, Maria was left to her own devices. Bored, she dropped out of school at age twelve and commenced work with a clothing manufacturer. Maria has a clear sense that people with disabilities were not just rejected; she was expected to 'overcome' her disability by conforming as best she could with prescribed behaviours. These behaviours were that one lip-reads and speaks. Sign language was not allowed even though a near relative was deaf and utilized what appears to be a system of family signs. The moral responsibility for Maria fell to her family. When she could fit in again, she could participate. Until then, Maria was their responsibility. These are the social consequences of deafness for Maria and her family.

Such families achieve a sense of coherency and continuity by situating an understanding of impairment within a discourse that requires the children or young people to 'overcome' their disability by conforming as best they can with certain practices. These behaviours are (again) that one lip-reads and speaks. When Deafened people cannot conform with such requirements, they pay the consequences:

> Well, let's just say that, em, over the years, my relatives have been pretty funny. Now I don't know whether this is because our parents could have rebuffed any attempt to talk about it or try and understand what's been going on, but whenever we used to go to parties or something like that, um, it was always assumed that oh! Jan can't socialize so stick her in the kitchen. We'll serve food, she can look after the drinks – no problem! So it's getting so that I haven't been to a, um, anything like that for years. (Jan)

Jan is not merely isolated; she has been marginalized. For the moment the notion of marginality can be taken somewhat literally in that Jan has been pushed to the fringes of the social interaction under consideration. However, marginality in the context of the experience of disability has a fuller meaning that I develop in this text. This meaning centres on the process and outcomes of interactions in which taken-for-granted *normalizing tendencies* are contested by the lived experience of deafness.

Bourdieu (1992) points out that the values and practices of an education system tell a lot about the society in question. Included within these values is the emphasis given to the system of language which is taught.

Lane (1993) remarks that the purpose of oral education has been to supplement the limitations of individualizing medical processes:

> The job of the educator is not to educate; it is to find an educational treatment for what the otologist and audiologist could not treat, the child's failure to acquire English normally. A difference has been identified, now a massive campaign begins to eradicate it. (p. 25)

The expectation that one must participate in the education system on the terms of hearing people facilitates the marginalization of deafened young people at school. The social consequences of impairment (reduced friendships, family problems and enforced isolation) are now evident. Jan's memories of her high-school dance bring the issue into focus:

> I can remember my grade 10 formal. You never believe what some people try. OK so we went out with my mum. My mum was extremely reluctant. We brought my dress. It was beautiful. Shoes, got my hair done, make-up whatever – I'm sorry, I didn't laugh then but I giggle now. I mean I just giggle at the actions of the people involved. Anyway, my aunt, they were getting guys from [...] and one other school. And my aunt worked in the library at [...]. They collared that poor guy who was supposed to partner me and said, don't worry about Jan, she's deaf, she lip reads, she's OK, she won't hurt you, she won't bite. He didn't show up! ... No, I was OK, I had fun, I had friends at school, but I remember coming home so devastated because, and that's when mum told me that they warned him about me. Well they didn't tell him, they warned him.

At school, respondents recall experiences of being neglected by the teachers for being too smart, too dumb or too something. In classrooms which privileged hearing people, it was impossible for deafened students to follow discussions as they bounced around the room or when teachers spoke as they faced the board. The absence of accessible communication environments locked respondents out of the curriculum and from the school process. Students who succeeded really had to work for it:

> I've had to work twice as hard ... to achieve the same results. (Jan)

The social world of the Deafened young person essentially consists of family and school networks. It is within the family that some sense of onset must be made. It is at school that the social consequences of loss are intensely encountered.

Sudden onset

Jeff was profoundly deafened as a result of an accident. He lives at home and is supported by his girlfriend, family and other friends. Following his accident, Jeff began a rehabilitation programme which was co-ordinated by a rehabilitation advocate. His rehabilitation programme consisted mainly of assessments and advice on the nature and range of communication skills and technologies available to him. Jeff taught himself to lip-read, noting that services which did exist for profoundly deaf people focused primarily on supporting people who were members of the Deaf Community:

> my main thing is just lip-reading because all of my friends here really haven't concentrated too much on sign language so, I'll pick things up one way or the other.

Jeff participates as a Deafened person in a hearing world on hearing terms. Tolerance and acceptance are extended to him by his networks, which realize that communication is now more difficult for him:

> All the people in the Church, they were really good ... everyone's really good, usually, on a whole. Most people went out of their way a bit to help you because they realized that it's a little bit harder.

The manual nature of Jeff's work means that deafness is not a barrier to earning a living. The management of workplace communication was facilitated by the advocate who investigated technical and practical solutions to communication difficulties as they arose. This resulted in the provision of a portable paging system, paid for by a workplace rehabilitation programme.

As a result of meningitis, Paul went deaf overnight. Married with children, the rapid onset of his hearing loss meant Paul, his wife Suzanne, his family, networks and workplace had to re-evaluate their relationships in order to achieve a sense of coherence and continuity. Suzanne remarks:

> I remember my parents came to pick me up; take me home. And when I told them about it and said you know Paul's deaf and he's going to be deaf forever sort of thing. It then started to hit me, and I started to think, what, what does this mean? What does it mean for him? What does it mean for me? What does it mean for the family?

Paul had a professional job that did not require continuous contact with the public or use of the telephone. Nonetheless, his job security did come into crisis and Suzanne had to negotiate part of the transition on his behalf. Once this crisis was over, work people were supportive and life went on. But communication remained difficult for Paul in all aspects of life. A level of continuity and coherence was achieved, but it was less than ideal. As Suzanne remarks, it could have been worse:

> Like if he lost his job he would have been dependent on me. And things would have been very different ... There's that social support, that work support – that recognition within the community that these people are people first – not somebody – not a disability. And I don't think this is any different from all the other you know – disabilities.

Gradual onset

For many people, acquired profound hearing loss arrives after a period of gradual onset. Unlike Jeff, there comes a time in the process of being deafened that one moves beyond difficult communication encounters which can be artfully managed. To engage the social means to linger near or within the borders of marginalization. For those who have been deafened for some time, the opportunity for marginalization was intensified by the large body aids and ear lugs once commonly available. Such aids typified the stereotype of impairment as uncontested abnormality rather than contested difference. Recalling wearing such devices, Ellen 'elected' to go through school with few if any friends, 'content' with her own company, pursuing isolated hobbies into adulthood:

> History and museum work and type of things I'm interested in does not appeal. Well, it may appeal to some individuals, but I haven't met any deaf people that are interested in the same things that I am interested in.

Ellen describes herself as a young person content in her own company. Deafened at age four, deafness was so much a part of Ellen's life that it is perceivable that living in a world with little communication was the norm for her. The distance between the onset and the outcome of acquired hearing loss has been so long, that a particular way of being is now normal life – being alone, doing things alone. Carol remarks in a similar fashion: 'I was the bookworm. So I sort of shied away from people, all that sort of thing.'

Later onset

People who are deafened later in life realize that able-bodiness forms part of a morally sanctioned bargain which they unwittingly established with people close to them and the broader community. The onset of deafness produces a breakdown of this bargain – it sets it aside. In the old arrangement, the 'normality' of the Hearing world – of hearing and speech – was part of the taken-for-granted agreement. A responsibility exists for the deafened individual and those close to them, to repair the breach as quickly as possible. This responsibility is highlighted in Parsons's (1951) notion of the 'sick role'. One is left alone to learn how to communicate, to cope with changes in family, work and social life, personal identity and professionals:

> The big thing I can remember is utter confusion! Not knowing what's happened. What you can see you can accept quickly but when it comes to hearing – because you can't see what's happening – the brain takes a long, long time to accept what's happened. Plus people round you don't accept that something's changed. It must be due to this problem and the truth is – you're the problem. You pick up vibes – this caused a lot of confusion. And of course a lot of stress. But when you['re] confused and over-stressed you're less likely to address properly and it takes a lot longer. I'd say they've been dreadful to me. (Sandra)

Those who experience rapid onset have the partial benefit of being thrust into an impairment management programme which serves as a de facto rite of passage. The process of managing acute injury signals to people that something has changed. The presence of a physical sign, such as a bandaged head, indicates to people that a change process is necessary and legitimate even if it is not understood. The experience of living with acquired profound hearing loss is not readily understood: 'It's hard for everybody, it's a hard concept, because they don't know what it's like' (Jeff). When the Deafened person is identified as the focus of the problem, the personal consequences of acquired profound hearing loss can be very high:

> My first husband was the type of person who refused to repeat himself. Refused to open his mouth. And when I went totally deaf he couldn't cope with it at all. He wouldn't face me. He wouldn't write anything down. It was all my fault. And um it got to the stage where he just gave up and I just gave up and we just broke up. He couldn't handle it. (Liz)

Once again it is the effect, rather than the extent of hearing loss, which is pivotal. This respondent's husband *should* have understood her problems as he was deaf in one ear and his mother also had severe hearing problems. But he did not. Liz's husband expected her to behave as though she did not have a hearing impairment. They attended parties and pressure was placed on Liz to return to work. Managing a severe hearing impairment within a social setting can be very tiring and stressful. For Liz it was particularly so. In time, Liz's husband left her for another woman of the same name. It was the final blow:

> He never came back ... but my doctor's helped me a lot. I still packed up I suppose. I had to go onto anti-depressant tablets for a long, long time. But I've got over it now.

It was the consequences of hearing impairment, that is Liz's marriage breakdown or at least the accumulation of a series of negative events that precipitated depression, not necessarily the hearing loss in itself. In Liz's case the onus for continuity and coherency falls upon the Deafened person. It is seen as his or her responsibility to enable social life to continue without disruption, or to experience marginalization as a consequence.

Recall the experiences of Jeff, Paul, Jan and Jean. They all experienced sudden onset of hearing loss, were the subjects of nurturing relationships as men and/or young people, and/or had access to an advocate. Liz has none of these supports but had to rely on her doctor and the pills he prescribed for her. Consider a further contrast for a moment; of two seemingly differing experiences. Liz, whose husband rejects her and Fiona (described below), whose husband controls her. In each situation, the hearing partner achieves coherency and continuity either by replacing their deafened partner or by making them communicate on their terms.

Fiona's story indicates the extent to which a person may need to go in order to sustain a relationship. Fiona lost her hearing suddenly as a result of the iatrogenic effects of a prescribed medication taken for a life-threatening illness. Fiona took the medication in full knowledge of what the consequences would be for her hearing. The impact of hearing loss on her life was substantial. An A grade sports player, Fiona could no longer play due to her loss of balance, and social encounters became problematic:

> I didn't go visiting, I wouldn't talk to anyone. And if I saw someone coming towards me in the street and I thought they were going to talk to me, I walk the other way because you say beg your pardon and if you don't get it the second time, say beg your pardon again, I used to just panic.

Fiona's ad hoc rehabilitation process was driven by the sense of inevitability which overcame her life, that there were no options but to learn to cope and get on with life. Fiona's partner had a very strong sense of what was normal and expectable. He organized Fiona into a disciplined regime of lip-reading and speech, for her own good. Fiona recalls the time:

> Fiona: When I first went deaf, I couldn't lip-read. They tried to teach me before I went deaf and I couldn't lip-read. I used to write things down on a slate. *Joe* threw it in the fire. They said look, if you don't learn, if you're gonna write everything down, you'll never ever ...
> Joe: I was pretty hard
> Fiona: That's how I've just had to survive, I had to learn to lip-read
> Joe: It was cruel, but I had to do it.

It is evident that the negotiation of changes to the daily practice of communication is not a straightforward exercise. Indeed, the notion of negotiation suggests that the facilitation of communicative changes is simply a matter of interpersonal skill. Fulcher (1993) points out that when communication is conceptualized in this manner, the 'moral and political aspects of action' (p. 23) are suppressed. In this instance, Joe's position is legitimated by the intersection of several *normalizing processes* (Foucault, 1991a; Fulcher, 1993). First, Joe asserted his power as the head of the household. It was his responsibility to be tough on Fiona, to make her accept her responsibilities. Second, the nature of Fiona's responsibilities were understood within an operationalization of a sense of 'normal' where normal meant that people hear and speak. Joe's position had a taken-for-granted validity that undermined the lived experience of being deafened. The adoption of practices and therefore the shaping of personal identity are influenced by the legitimacy afforded to particular techniques for managing the body in everyday life. Identity development is therefore a political process too.

Adrian experienced slow onset and was supported by an 'understanding' wife, who had since died. He could lip-read extremely well and he had come to accept a life of relative isolation outside of work. Since he retired, his personal networks have been sustained to a limited extent by visiting nearby families. He is able to hear enough to enjoy his hobby of writing music, which he shares as a common interest with his son. This seems to sustain him as he is able to participate in his existing networks. He has not lost everything. He lingers on the edge but has not as yet fallen over – not yet experienced that fatal threshold shift that makes all the difference between being in and being out of the hearing world.

Gender also influences the acceptability of deafness and the assistance offered. The community is prepared to gather around and support males in ways that are not extended to Deafened women. On the one hand, there is an assumption about managing illness that implies that women ought to be able to cope with such crises and get on with their life. On the other hand, there is also an assumption that men need assistance to re-establish themselves within roles such as work – a theme to which I shall return below.

Acquired profound hearing loss also disrupts the coherency and threatens the continuity of one's relationships as a (grand)parent. For some it means never hearing their (grand)children speak to them. When a parent is deafened, the children are left to cope as best they can with a loss of intimacy as well. Sandra recalls:

> for instance, if my son at one stage – my daughter would talk, talk, talk, talk and finally it would penetrate my mind that somebody's talking to me. And I'd turn and ask her to repeat. But my son would say it once. And that was it. And sometime there I was washing dishes once, busy washing the dishes, he was about three, four, he stood behind me and said something and stood there and waited and waited and waited. The only thing I knew was about, the first I knew

> about it was when suddenly I felt the floor vibrate, it was wooden. He'd thrown himself down in a tantrum because Mum was ignoring him. My husband would never tell them that mummy's ears don't work – tap her. He'd refuse to; he'd sit back with his arms folded. That day, I turned around to find a mouth full of abuse being hurled at me, because I ignore the kids all the time. (Sandra)

The onset of hearing loss demanded the renegotiation of relationships and identities by all partners to the interaction. Liz's husband was not prepared to negotiate and left. Sandra's husband passively and actively resisted any challenge to his taken-for-granted assumptions about the phonocentric nature of his lifestyle and facilitated his children's resistance to it as well. Renegotiation means that Deafened people have to re-establish their sense of identity in practical situations that are informed by competing discourses. It is not just about feeling or being different – it is about the exercise of power in daily practice. It is about acting differently and having to decide whether or not one will contest practices which may marginalize and suppress the lived experience of being Deafened. Acquired profound hearing loss thrusts the Deafened person into a borderland. Friends and family have the option to decide whether or not they will share in the experience of living in multiple and at times, seemingly illegitimate worlds. Anzaldua (1987) describes the experience of living in a borderland:

> Living on borders and in margins, keeping intact one's shifting and multiple identity and integrity, is like trying to swim in a new element, an alien element ... And yes, the 'alien' element has become familiar – never comfortable, not with society's clamour to uphold the old, to rejoin the flock, to go with the herd. No, not comfortable, but home. (Gunew and Yeatman, 1993: 218)

Thus coherency and continuity, as a sense of being at home with one's self and circumstance, need to be worked out within a context which often requires the Deafened person to 'overcome' their impairment and its social consequences by conforming with certain prescribed behaviours that are consistent with existing forms of able-bodied family life. The practices associated with this discourse seek to 'dissolve' (Fulcher, 1993: 10) the experience of difference by *disintegrating* the existence of deafness through the imposition of communication via the modes of hearing and speech. Deafness as difference is not only contested by a discourse concerned with assimilating Deafened people into hearing culture, the practices associated with this discourse refuse to provide a forum in which an identity developed through communicative practice can be negotiated. Within this text I utilize the phrases communicative practice or communicative action. The phrase is intended to be read literally. It is not an appropriation of Habermas's (1990) *communicative action*. Continuity and coherency may be negotiated in a manner which enables the Deafened people to reintegrate themselves in networks that they value, wherein the everyday behaviours of hearing culture are not taken as given. However, it appears that a degree of advocacy and support is required, at least in the initial phases of negotiation as meaning systems are contested and (in)validated.

Initial negotiations take place in conjunction with partners and family members for whom support or advice services are all but non-existent. There are also no specific marriage and family counselling or similar support services that are readily accessible for Deafened people. Only the voluntary agencies offer any counselling services. For the most part, these services are provided by volunteers with little training, within the frameworks of charity-based, tragedy-centred programmes or poorly resourced, self-help movements. In the course of the research behind this text, 38 people were interviewed concerning the impact of deafness in their lives. Of these, 18 people report at least one relationship break-up associated either with the process of the onset of hearing loss or following onset. Undisrupted relationships were associated with longstanding or less disruptive onsets. Those in longer-term relationships tended to have met their partners after onset. Those deafened, whose relationships stayed together, indicated that although severe losses may cause strain on relationships, the extent of the strain appears to be managed, at least to the point of not completely destroying the relationship. Personal networks may be sustained on a daily basis by the combined effect of participants in such networks being prepared to change aspects of speaking and hearing so that communication and/or tasks can be achieved. However, the cost of participation is high and compromise results:

> at this stage in life to break up, doesn't really help the family and you lose your home and everything, ye roots are down. I've put up with him. (Sandra)

By now, the reader may have also noted the Anglo-Saxon pseudonyms I have employed in relating respondents' experiences. This is no accident. Only two respondents were from non-English-speaking backgrounds and both spoke English. The fact is that there are very few ethnic-specific or bilingual services for Deafened people in countries like Australia. If one cannot speak English, then access to assistance will be extremely difficult.

Work

Deafness is perceived as a barrier to effective participation in the workplace. This perception arises because the workplace privileges telecommunication systems such as the telephone and the television over video-conferencing, video-telephones, telephone typewriters, electronic mail, facsimile and paging systems. Of course, this is slowly changing. Nonetheless, deafness is not accepted as a legitimate barrier to participation. One is expected and indeed needs to overcome such barriers in order to gain employment; but, as Sandra observes, 'you can't participate because you don't know what is being said'. Employment options are limited to the tasks that one can perform unaided. Little accommodation on the part of the employer is considered reasonable or necessary. Once again, change processes need to be considered beyond simplistic conceptions of negotiation that assume that disabled people are in a position to negotiate with equal power.

Christine had slow onset hearing loss. When her hearing finally disappeared (along with her husband and job working directly with the public), she was left to support her children. She describes the experience of trying to get a job:

> (Sigh) But I couldn't go back to [my old job] because of the communication problem ... so I had to look at other options. I could type. Computers were starting to come out then. I had a problem with the phone. A lot of clerical jobs are very phone-oriented. I couldn't get to a phone, I was living in [town] at the time. They had no relay service. No TTYs or anything like that. So I took to door-knocking. It took me about three weeks of door-knocking. I went around to all the companies and asked if they had any vacancies, and why I had come to them [and] what I was looking for. And I struck it lucky with someone who had a relative who was deaf [and] had a hearing problem. So I got the job. I stayed there for five years. And that's how I supported myself and family.

Christine got a job doing bookkeeping and other clerical tasks. Christine got lucky because her employer understood deafness and allowed it to be encompassed within the bounds of legitimacy. Most Deafened people are not so lucky. They encounter specific structural barriers when seeking employment. Let us take a moment to examine these. First, Deafened adults tend to have lower educational qualifications than the rest of the community (Table 2.1). This may be due in part to the impact of undetected hearing loss beginning onset while people are still at school.

Table 2.2 lists respondents' employment status for those in paid work, showing that the majority of those in paid work have full-time jobs. Table 2.3 provides a comparison of workforce participation rates for Deafened adults as compared with all Australians. It can be seen that for both groups (implantees and non-implantees) workforce participation rates compare well with the national average for those in the younger age groups, but the rate falls dramatically for those aged over 55 years.

Table 2.1: Highest education level attained for people aged 65 years or less (N = 143; missing = 2)

	Implantees	*Non-implantees*	*Total*	*Australia*
No school education	1 (1.0%)	1 (2.5%)	2 (1.4%)	
Still at school	2 (2.0%)	1 (2.5%)	3 (2.1%)	
Primary education	8 (7.9%)	3 (7.5%)	11 (7.8%)	5.4%
Some high school	35 (34.7%)	16 (40.0%)	51 (36.2%)	36.3%
Completed high school (yr 12)	25 (24.8%)	6 (15.0%)	31 (22.0%)	17.9%
Some post-school training	16 (15.8%)	5 (12.5%)	21 (14.9%)	8.8%
Completed qualification	14 (13.9%)	8 (20.0%)	22 (15.6%)	31.5%*
Total	101 (71.6%)	40 (28.4%)	141 (100%)	100%

*Includes skilled vocational and trades qualifications.
Comparative source: Australian Bureau of Statistics (1999: 285) Persons aged 16–64, by educational attainment, May 1997.

Table 2.2: Amount of paid work undertaken by those employed (aged 65 years or less)

	Implantees	*Non-implantees*	*Total*
Full-time	36 (73.5%)	15 (78.9%)	51 (75.0%)
Part-time	10 (20.4%)	4 (21.1%)	14 (20.6%)
Casual	3 (6.1%)	0	3 (4.4%)
Total	49	19	68 (100%)

Table 2.3: Workforce participation rate for people aged 64 years or less (n = 135)

	Implantees		*Non-implantees*		*Australia*
	In workforce	Not in workforce	In workforce	Not in workforce	
< 55 yrs	53 (76.8%)	16 (23.2%)	24 (80.0%)	6 (20.0%)	78.6
56–64 yrs	10 (35.7%)	18 (64.3%)	3 (37.5%)	5 (62.5%)	48.1
Total	63 (56.3%)		27 (58.8%)		67.4

Comparative source: Labour force participation rates, by age and birthplace, Australian Bureau of Statistics, September 1998, Cat 6203.0 p. 29.

The average age of deafened people of working age are approximately 48.6 years (s.d. 11.6 years). Between one-third and a half of each group reported being in paid employment (with the male rate of employment being higher) with 72 per cent of these reporting being in full-time employment (Table 2.4).

Table 2.4: Occupation status for those in paid work (n = 68; people aged 65 years or less)

	Implantees	*Non-implantees*	*Total*	*Australia (%)*
Manager/self-employed	11 (22.4%)	4 (21.1%)	15 (22.1%)	7.5
Professional	11 (22.4%)	1 (5.3%)	12 (17.6%)	17.5
Para-professional	4 (8.2%)	0	4 (5.9%)	10.4
Trade	7 (14.3%)	3 (15.8%)	10 (14.7%)	13.6
Clerical	5 (10.2%)	4 (21.1%)	9 (13.2%)	4.6
Sales/service	0	1 (5.3%)	1 (1.5%)	16.9
Production/transport/ plant/labour	2 (4.0%)	3 (15.8%)	5 (7.4%)	10.3
Other	9 (18.4%)	3 (15.8%)	12 (17.6%)	0
Total	49 (72.1%)	19 (27.9%)	68 (100%)	100

Comparative source: Australian Bureau of Statistics (1999: 23) Employed persons by occupation, Annual average 1997–98.

It can be seen from Tables 2.4 and 2.5 that Deafened adults are comparatively less well educated than the general population and are concentrated within trades and unskilled employment. The higher number of Deafened people working in professions in this data set reflects pre-onset qualifications coupled with the capacity of such employees to negotiate continued employment with minimal or supported contact with the public (e.g. accountancy). As a group, their employment status has essentially not changed from the work offered to deaf people one hundred years ago (see Winzer, 1993).

Table 2.5 presents data comparing average weekly earnings of Deafened people to that of the population. According to the Australian Bureau of Statistics' Survey on *Disability, Ageing and Carers* (1993b), 74 per cent of totally deaf people earn no more than $15,643 per annum. At this time, average household income for Australians was $27,500, indicating that Deafened people earn significantly less than most Australians.

What happens to people's employability when they lose their hearing? The answer remains unclear. However, respondents' experiences identify a number of trends. First, the impact of onset depends upon the type of work one does and the likely consequences arising for the person.

Table 2.5: Average weekly earnings for deafened people of working age by group (n = 143, missing = 17)

	Implantees (in paid work)	*Implantees (not in paid work)*	*Non-implantees (in paid work)*	*Non-implantees (not in paid work)*	*Total*
Earnings					
Less than average	29 (32%)	43 (34%)	16 (42%)	19 (50%)	107
Average	4 (5%)	1 (1%)	0	0	5
Above average	11 (13%)	0	3 (8%)	0	14
Total	44 (50%)	44 (50%)	19 (50%)	19 (50%)	126

Second, it depends upon the attitudes to deafness held by helping professionals and organizations who fund hearing rehabilitation services. Certainly people can get by without interventions such as cochlear implantation, but is *getting by* a sufficient outcome? Let us examine this question in the light of case-study material. In Jeff's situation (discussed earlier), deafness made little difference to his employability. For others, although onset may be diagnosed as severe to profound, one is able to retain lifelong employment, even if it is not in a preferred area. Adrian moved between a variety of retail jobs while his hearing was sufficient for face-to-face or telephone communication. He relied heavily on lip-reading, and was able to do his job. Roger's hearing deteriorated to the point that he could no longer conduct a number of his supervisor duties. He describes how his workmates accommodated his loss:

> I was senior postman and early in the morning had to ring up. Sometimes the bag would come from the wrong area. We were at [town] and we had bags that went to [another town] and different places and I had to ring up. I had to get one of the other blokes – I couldn't hear too well. That was when I was about er ... I s'pose about 60.

However, unlike Roger and Jeff, there comes a time with acquired profound hearing loss where informal accommodation in itself is insufficient and job redesign or retraining needs to be considered or the person must leave the workforce. Gena, a health professional with daily patient contact, was confronted with this situation and withdrew from employment:

> And then I was working at the time and I carried on for quite along time ... it became more and more difficult. And eventually I couldn't take telephone calls, although I had staff to do that for me. But there were some situations where it would have been much better if I could have done it myself, but I couldn't do that. And eventually I had to give up work all together.

The issue of retraining or redeployment in other areas of work was not considered.

Similarly, two male teachers who acquired severe hearing loss eventually ceased employment. Both had access to superannuation-based disability pensions. For one, the work changes associated with his deafness became a positive factor in his life, while for the other, it was deemed negative. For the first respondent, potential negative personal consequences of acquired hearing loss were not apparent in his life because he chose, for reasons other than deafness, to disrupt his personal networks completely and to work to re-establish himself within the Gay community. It may be that the onset of hearing loss provided him with the opportunity to make changes he had been contemplating for some time. However, had his employer's insurer not been prepared to allow him to go on to a disability payment scheme, he would have been in very different circumstances, and life may not have been so wonderful. He would have had to try for a state disability pension or more likely, go on unemployment benefits. There was no apparent reason that prevented this respondent from being retrained to run a school for deaf children or to undertake a programme of occupational retraining. But such options were not seriously considered:

> [I] saw the psychologist who ran a whole bank of tests and all the general carry on and eventually said 'well, yes I can see you've got a problem' and the Principal [of his school] backed that up and I had to go to my own doctor and I had to go to my specialist – got medical stuff from them. Basically, I was in the situation where the Principal said 'You've been doing an excellent job, but at an increasing cost to yourself and I don't think it's fair on you – it's time the Department took some responsibility and did something about this'. My own doctor said 'I'm not an educationist, but as far as I'm concerned, I'm aware that there's a problem and I've sent you off to a specialist', which I've been doing ever since I've had mumps anyway. And as the specialist said, 'I'm not an educationalist, I'm willing to give a specialist's report, but I'm not prepared to say you shouldn't be teaching'.

The Education Department's preparedness to allow this employee redundancy on medical grounds reflects a narrowly constructed view of the abilities of Deafened people and understates the capabilities of aural and occupational rehabilitation services. In addition, the pension option cannot be considered cost-effective from the insurers' perspective, but reflects their general lack of awareness of hearing rehabilitation services.

The second teacher was devastated by having to stop work, despite having recourse to a disability pension. The sense of devastation related to his loss of professional and personal networks. Following hearing loss and other health problems, his family relocated when his wife found employment. In his old networks he was remembered as a teacher who had gone deaf; in his new networks, he was the deaf partner of a professional woman. Although he also retained hearing and speech communication, it was with greater difficulty than the first teacher. Specifically, he had no basis upon which to engage new networks other than from what he considered to be a wholly negative standpoint.

Further research is required into the area of employment, deafness and access to rehabilitation. But before closing this section several final points are noted. First, the workforce participation rate for Deafened adults falls dramatically for people aged over 55 years. The data indicates that the majority of these people leave work early *because* of their deafness (see Chapter 8 on enhancing employment outcomes for further details on this). Second, Deafened adults earn significantly less than the rest of the population. This may in part be due to the (pre-deafness) occupational status of individuals, but it may also be due to discriminatory factors operating in the workplace that require attention. Given the reasonably high number of Deafened people in the workplace, it is feasible that a glass ceiling effect is in operation. A glass ceiling effect refers to the phenomenon wherein people's advancement in the workplace is blocked because of discriminatory attitudes and behaviours.

Addressing the disadvantageous social position of Deafened adults is very important. As I have shown elsewhere (Hogan et al., 2000), a person's health-related quality of life is correlated with employment, education and socio-economic well-being. It is critical therefore that rehabilitation programmes address the socio-economic factors addressing their clients, not simply their auditory needs.

Framing the issue

Why should a non-life-threatening, physiological change in a bodily organ no larger than the nail of the little finger have such ramifications for both deafened individuals and those close to them? Irrespective of when the onset of deafness occurs in a person's life, its impact is profoundly social. Yet it is the individual who has become deafened who is configured as dysfunctional in social interactions. The interaction itself is not. The site of difference is located within an individual body, but its impact can only be established within that body's social relations. Deafness demands a change in behaviour which throws into dispute every person's taken-for-granted rules about the conduct of everyday life (Foucault, 1988). This conflict between the individual, the broader community and differing perceptions of what constitutes proper behaviour impacts, in a very real way, on the lives of Deafened people. So it is important to stand back for a moment and consider this impact in some detail.

CHAPTER 3

Carving out a space to act: acquired impairment and contested identity

Preamble

We have seen so far that acquired profound hearing loss can have an enormous impact on the life of the Deafened person. We have also seen that the negative consequences associated with disability arise because of the way society has understood disability – primarily as a deficit within the body of the individual that results in social dependencies that communities have in turn sought to eliminate through various means. Now we know that even with advanced hearing aids and cochlear implants, impairment is still part of the Deafened person's life. Even those who do very well with the implant are soon disabled by a broken cable or a flat battery. Nonetheless, it would be simplistic to suggest that all the problems faced by Deafened people would disappear if the rest of the community simply picked up its attitude, became more tolerant and learnt to communicate better. Even in the best of possible worlds, such social change is two generations away. By the same token much can be done to enable clients to achieve satisfactory interpersonal relationships through the implementation of appropriate rehabilitation programmes. But before we set off into a discussion about what an 'appropriate' programme might entail, it is necessary to develop our understanding of the interpersonal dynamics confronting Deafened people and those with whom they share their lives.

In this chapter I explore the issue of identity development as a social as well as an individual phenomenon. Within the individualized medical model of disability, it might be suggested that following the onset of impairment, one has to go through various stages of grieving before one 'comes to terms' with disability. To a degree this is true. Yet coming to terms with disability is also about recognizing and learning to deal with the dreadful manner in which western society treats disabled people; of recognizing that many of society's nasty hidden messages now actually refer to one's self. One's sense of who I am and ideas and strategies for surviving in the world now that one has a disability, are obviously developed in one's mind, but such development takes place in relation to those people and institutions who now make up one's life. The psychosocial adjustment process is about coming to terms *with* and, to differing degrees, accepting or rejecting the dominant discourse. But this is not something that just occurs inside one's head – it actually happens with other people because adjustment to disability is as much about taking on new skills, behaviours and technologies as it is about attitude development. Behavioural and psychological adjustment occur in tandem within the social networks that make up one's life. One of the key barriers faced by Deafened people within the adjustment process is developing a repertoire of skills, attitudes, behaviours and technologies that work for them both in the technical as well as the social sense.

People want to be able to talk to someone other than their mother – no matter how nice she might be! Identity development is therefore as much a psychosocial, as it is a technological, issue. In this chapter we explore how several Deafened adults have spontaneously developed their deafness identity and worked through the adjustment process. We will see that when individuals are left within the individualizing medical approach, the adjustment process is stressful, painful and isolating. But we also learn that there are alternatives to this negative outcome. Once these lessons are recognized, we can then move on to planning our interventions so that much of this pain can be minimized, and outcomes optimized.

> embodiment ... cannot be unproblematically taken as the logical or defining feature of the person or of personal identity through time. Attributes of personhood, such as the continuity and coherence of the person through time, are socially and culturally established, they are not merely given in the physical fact of embodiment. Self identity is thus something that has to be established socially through a set of discourses which are discursive and practical. (Moore, 1994)

Introduction

Communication based on hearing and speech are part of taken-for-granted rules for daily practice. The nature of these practices structure social participation and access to culture. If language structures practice, then a subjectivity centred on deafness, on the absence of the prescribed mode of interaction, means that an individual is unable to participate in a manner expected within the social. Spoken and written language shape the core of everyday interactions to which most are accustomed. Of course, the rules of interaction governed by communication go far beyond syntax; within communication are the prescribed rules for the everyday. Acceptance, humour, anger, rejection: these are all communicated by sounds, through intonation, speed, emphasis and silence. Language constitutes people as very specific types of actors. The governance of deafness is about shaping behaviour so that the core rules and values of hearing culture and the systems, technologies and networks that sustain it, can be secured and upheld in very specific ways.

The onset of profound hearing loss disrupts daily practice for Deafened individuals and those with whom they interact. This disruption is not just about communication; it is about deeply held values concerning the social position of people with disabilities where disability is perceived as a personal deficit and a moral failing. The onset of disability signals a massive change in a person's social position and constitutes a personal crisis for the individual. Identity as a social phenomenon becomes apparent as individuals are perceived by themselves and others as different; an experience of difference that goes beyond Goffman's notions of stigma (1963; for a critique on stigma see Finkelstein, 1980). The lived experience of being deaf contests the notion that it is a hearing world. People who acquire a profound hearing loss find themselves acting within a new context based upon old frameworks for meaningful practice. They enter a world turned upside down by actors, embodied and institutional, who set out to (re)shape the nature, meaning and trajectory of the experience at hand. As any Deafened person struggles with the idea of *what shall I do?* now that I am deaf, they do so within the context of their own historicity. (The nature, meaning and trajectory of life for people born deaf is also contested by ableist society. However, the process is different. People born into families of Deaf people join a community where the right to be deaf is validated and supported. People born deaf into hearing families face similar challenges to those of Deafened adults. However, in their case, decisions about culture and identity are often made for them by others; a decision that many may seek to reverse in adult life.)

> identity stems from agency, and presupposes a continuity of practices with respect to historical conditions of existence. (Warren, 1988: 199)

Acting in this context is about reconciling changes (1) in the lived experience of social relations, (2) within available conceptual frameworks, (3) managed within a context of being acted upon as well as acting, (4) while trying to re-establish some direction in life; a direction that reflects some notion of 'normality'.

Learning to live with deafness is a work of personal reformation shaped by competing systems of meaning, social production and power

(Foucault, 1988). Within the seemingly innocent walls of our hearing rehabilitation clinics, an intense power struggle takes place. Whether we like it or not, within our clinics, we exercise power. This power results from the synergistic efforts of various agencies (government, insurers, technology manufacturers, professional groups of doctors and therapists, self-help groups). Sawicki (1991) points out that power, from Foucault's perspective is neither centralized nor repressive. Rather, power results because institutions and individuals work together in order to produce something. The primary objective of hearing clinics is not the elimination or suppression of Deaf culture, but the reproduction of Deafened people as hearing people. The minds of Deafened people and in turn their bodies are the sites upon which this power is exercised. Here I examine how Deafened people engage such technological processes as they seek to renegotiate an identity as a Deafened person where their legitimacy to do so may be contested and where decisions may be made without access to the full range of choices available. To achieve this end, the experiences of three people, Carol, Sandra and Jan, are described and their process of engagement from three view points are considered as they seek to retain an identity as hearing people and to create a dual identity, with or without the use of various technologies.

Acquired profound hearing loss

Deafened people share a number of common experiences. Generally speaking they are born with some useful hearing, acquire speech and develop an identity as able-bodied people. The time hearing loss occurs may vary from early childhood to late adult life. Yet irrespective of the time of onset, deafness projects the Deafened person into a marginal social position. The extent of this marginality is dependent on the extent to which the individual retains usable hearing and speech skills. Practices associated with the notion of stigma management can be taken on by the Deafened individual because the ableist discourse holds that the inability to communicate in various settings is a sign of personal failure. ('Ableist is a political term used by people with disabilities to call attention to assumptions made about normalcy' (Davis, 1995: 172)). This is not, of course, the sign of complete failure; community attitudes to deafness have shaped attitudes in such a fashion that complete failure has been stereotyped in those who use sign language. The discourse reminds Deafened people that they are right to be embarrassed by their inability to converse in a fluent manner, but while they remain above the 'feral' pit of signing, they can retain some sense of dignity.

A silence overshadows the experience of disability when it is construed within notions of stigma and shame. This silence skips over the difficulty of surviving a marginalizing process. It is a silence Deafened people have to endure and from which many seek to escape.

Carol

Carol acquired impaired hearing in stages, beginning with a childhood illness and culminating in a final loss in early adulthood. At 18 she acquired her first hearing aid. Carol describes her childhood as shy and socially isolated (the bookworm), but as though she had chosen this path. The onset of hearing loss is often slow and progressive. This transitional process 'locks' the individual into a trajectory that is not interrupted by the onset of total deafness. Rather, the direction of the trajectory is intensified. Following the complete loss of hearing, one must work even harder to remake the self as a hearing person. It is here that the classical interpretation of Parson's (1951) 'sick role' is gathered into the morality surrounding acquired profound hearing loss. Within the sick role a moral obligation falls on the Deafened person to participate in prescribed rituals and disciplines in order to remake themselves as hearing people. Until they are remade, they cannot disengage. The reality, of course, is that the most profoundly Deafened people never regain the ease of communication they once knew and, in consequence, they are eternally *patients*. Nor are they considered normal, no matter how much they transform themselves. As such, an element of dehumanization remains.

Carol was ashamed of her deafened body to the point that she no longer wished to be seen by people. Deafness turned an adult experience of interaction into an experience of childhood – to be seen but not to hear. Warren (1988:148) aptly remarks that 'communication requires intelligibility and intelligence requires rule-following'. By inference, Deafened people become stupid because they are regarded as not having sufficient basic intelligence to participate properly in daily interactions. Carol's experience of self had been developed in the light of problematic social encounters, in the knowledge of the demands of communication environments – those already known and those anticipated in the future. Her sense of self was '... not just divided between the remembered and the forgotten, the future and the past, but between the self and the other' (Diprose, 1993: 9). Carol was very much aware of this dual process of who she was and was not. Reeling from marginalizing encounters, she remarked:

> I was becoming very much an introvert, that I was isolating myself from people. I didn't want to go places because I knew I couldn't talk to them and so forth.

Carol avoids the detail of such encounters: the *and so forth*. The *and so forth* encapsulates the marginalizing process, often described using

Goffman's (1963) notion of stigma and spoiled identity. The concept of stigma suggests that when people are confronted with the threat of marginalization, they may experience a sense of shame, guilt or anxiety because they recognize that they lack something or possess something considered by others to be undesirable. The stigma response, as it were, is thought to resolve awkward moments in otherwise 'normal' interactions. Giddens (1991: 66) says that 'shame often focuses on that "visible" [i.e. identifiable] aspect of self, the body' (my inclusion). Historically, deafness may have been socially visualized by people wearing identifiers such as hearing aids or cochlear implant speech processors. Modern hearing aids and 'discreetly' worn cochlear implant speech processors create a setting in which such identifiers may go undetected. Deafness is most commonly visualized when spoken social interaction breaks down and in so doing threatens to identify the Deafened person as other, and to disclose the gap (and all moral imperatives associated with it) inherent to deafness as a result of the medico-deficit model of the body.

Carol subsequently met other people who were in a similar situation. This group had developed skills and communication tactics generally found to be acceptable to hearing people. These tactics meant that one could essentially 'pass' as a hearing person. Carol's feelings about herself changed as did her social activities and networks:

> You didn't have to be embarrassed about having the hearing aid sticking [out of] your ear like this body aid, like this big ear piece here or cords showing and all that sort of thing.

Carol translated the communication ideas she learnt across various aspects of her life so that she could *pass* as a hearing person. For her it became a challenge to participate in the hearing world on their terms. Confronted with the slide into personal dissolution, Carol set off on a trajectory that was supported by an ideological framework and social process. Carol regarded herself as more fortunate than most – the little residual hearing she retained greatly aided her ability to lip-read and therefore 'pass' as a hearing person. Thus by behaving as a 'normal' hearing person, Carol was able to gain some control over an otherwise dehumanizing process. As such, passing offers a limited form of liberation because the Deafened person, via the adoption of particular behaviours, can pursue legitimated associations and their ensuing benefits.

The practical and symbolic techniques of personal understanding and formation promoted by the traditional hearing clinic sustain Deafened people within problematic social relations. These techniques include training Deafened people in the use of 'communication tactics' which consist of a range of strategies for manipulating the communication environment in order to maximize one's chance of hearing without disrupting the 'normal' flow of communication. Alternative pedagogies focus on developing a Deafened person's ability to communicate on a more equal basis, enabling individuals to renegotiate the rules of communication and social engagement. The privileged nature of hearing culture is not brought into question. By inference, the source of this problem is located within Deafened people and their attention is focused on developing coping strategies to fit in with the rest of the hearing world.

Not every Deafened person follows this path. In fact, it is possible for Deafened people to pursue alternative communication pathways and to validate their identity as Deafened people.

Sandra

> But I would not call myself deaf or fully hearing mind – somewhere in between the two which gets a little bit awkward. It's like sitting on a picket fence and it gets very uncomfortable. (Sandra)

Sandra was in upper primary school when her hearing started to deteriorate. Sandra quickly discovered the personal price of nonconformity with these rules and her world was in chaos. She could neither understand what was happening, nor do anything about it. It created an anger within her which she carries to this day – forty years later. The diagnosis of deafness did little to enhance Sandra's social position within the school environment. Lumbered with a large body aid, which amplified everything in the room, she was supposed to be able to cope in school just like any one else; reading the teacher's lips as the teacher wrote on the blackboard! Sandra's punishment for being deafened continued into adulthood. No one employed her. No one was prepared to accommodate her communication needs in a workplace which relied on telephone work. Luck briefly changed and Sandra was employed in a government department as a clerical worker. The position came about as a result of a programme of affirmative action targeting disabled people. But circles of oppression surrounded Sandra, as a Deafened person and as a woman. Being deaf, Sandra was not allowed to join the workplace superannuation fund nor would her insurance company cover her for driving a car. Sandra held her job for five years before being forced to resign because she got married – married women were not allowed to work in the public service in Australia until 1968. If school had not already strongly suggested to her that there was something very negative about being deaf, adult life confirmed the reality.

As her adult life progressed, Sandra's hearing sensitivity fluctuated – sometimes for the better, other times not. Unfortunately, the management of a fluctuating loss is not simply achieved by adjusting the volume of a hearing aid. Sandra's loss fluctuated by frequency as well as in intensity. Sandra had learnt to integrate visual stimuli with the little auditory input she had left, and this had been enough to enable her to communicate. When her losses fluctuated, so did her communication skills, until such time as she was able to recalibrate her ears, eyes and brain:

> But then I had the shocking confusion – a doorbell. Before I used to be able to hear through the hearing aid – it dings! Now I hear a bit of a 'thawong' – and I stand there and think – what's that? What's that? My mind couldn't connect that sound up. It was a totally different sound. There were other bits and pieces. Then I find I couldn't lip-read. I would look at the person, but I couldn't lip-read them. Nothing would go in. I have since read of a woman in America who had a stroke and lost her sound suddenly overnight too. Same thing happened ... her ability to lip-read also left her.

The fluctuation had additional consequences. Sandra's capacity to communicate would also fluctuate, and this meant that people would not know how to cope with her when her skills changed. Life took on a new level of chaos. Stress was everywhere. With her children, her husband and friends, confusion reigned. The loss of hearing not only constituted a loss of the self, but also a loss of intimacy with those near to her. The resulting chaos and incoherency was exacerbated by a medical profession that could only monitor the process. They could neither predict nor control the changes.

Despite the explosive, stress-filled unpredictability of home life, Sandra worked to maintain a 'normal' hearing family life. Sandra readily admits that it would have been easier for her to sign and to live as a Deaf person. For Sandra, the incoherency of 'being oral' (as she calls it) when you are deaf, does not work with little children. They cannot comprehend that one can talk but not hear. There were not and still are no services that facilitate families making the types of changes required by the onset of profound hearing loss. In Sandra's mind, this has amounted to a prejudice against a Deaf way of life. While Sandra persevered with hearing culture at home, she gradually discovered that there were other ways of being deaf.

Brought up within a hearing family, deafened at a young age, engaged in individualizing medicalized processes for many years and married in a hearing family, Sandra developed strong attachments with hearing culture. However, her constant engagement with marginalizing processes set her off on multiple pathways. Reflecting on the process she remarked: 'the isolation caused my mind to take that bearing towards the Deaf mind'.

What does Sandra mean by a 'Deaf mind' when her background is so steeped in hearing culture? Sandra collapsed forty years of change into a few sentences. It is important to unpack this silence, because it is so informative. Sandra complained that there were no signposts to tell the Deafened person how to cope, how to manage others, how to change others, or to tell others that they should change. For Sandra, there was not much use in talking to a hearing service provider about being Deaf – what did they know about the everyday encounters faced by Deafened people within a world hostile to the overall experience of disability? For Sandra, the adjustment process was one of constant adaptation to an unstable environment, in which one needed a lot of support. Looking forward, Sandra holds that such support is still required by Deafened people: 'they also need to be able to come in frequently and sit down and talk about the problems that happen with it – the hearing aid, for example – whether they [are] finding it makes their head feel its splitting apart'. But she goes further – future services must provide an empathic connection between the provider and service user, a connection that can only come from a meeting of minds, a unity born of common experience and understanding. For example, only a Deaf person can teach another how to listen to music through feeling the vibrations! Peer support provides a forum in which the problems of hearing culture can be worked through, strategies developed, problems resolved. It is not simply a matter of counselling but of interpersonal understanding about the overall change process in which the Deafened person has engaged and the mutual acceptance arising from a common road travelled. As Starr (1991: 29) remarks:

> [W]e are the ones who have done the invisible work of creating a unity of action in the face of a multiplicity of selves ...This experience is about multi-vocality or heterogeneity, but not only that. We are at once heterogeneous, split apart, multiple ... we have experience of a self unified only through action, work and the patchwork of collective biography.

Sandra has arrived at the point of having developed a Deaf mind over a long period of time. Even then, she points out that she lives in multiple worlds. Her family connections keep her firmly in the hearing world. Yet Sandra is far from being a 'pretend deaf person' (a phrase used within the Australian Deaf community to refer to people with acquired hearing loss, particularly mild to moderate losses; such people are not considered to be really deaf, particularly as they engage the community as hearing people and experience few, if any, of the disadvantages associated with being completely deaf). She is multi-modal: she signs, speaks and lip-reads. At home she uses a range of technologies including a telephone type-writer (TTY), and various visual alerts (e.g. flashing lights to know someone's at the door). But Sandra restates constantly the need for peer support and skills-building services for Deafened people and their families. If they had been available, her life would have been a lot less stressful, and her transition to a world of multiple identity would have occurred a lot earlier and certainly more smoothly. For Starr (1991), the legitimacy of the multiple self is reclaimed by validating the hidden work undertaken to remake the self as a Deafened person, by defying the construct of able-bodiment and through recognizing the benefits, the personal power and the marginality arising from living in multiple worlds. As Sandra demonstrates, the experience of the multiple self is real and can be achieved.

Phonocentric culture seeks to deter Deafened people from developing this multiple sense of identity, this capacity to exercise personal power; it presents it as a chasm, an abyss to be avoided:

> The big problem with the hearing person (who) goes deaf is they have been brought up with the idea that the Deaf are weird and they're frightened of moving over there. Frightened of going out on their own, frightened of having their own foundations torn up. There is still a need to bridge that gap – and it is important to still operate in the hearing world – but you are under stress ... You've got to battle to bridge that gap yourself – so there's a real need for ... people to try to move towards the deaf world, for their own good. The more they can relax, the better they cope, plus you find yourself as a person of some worth. (Sandra)

Sandra recognizes the experience of deficit endured by Deafened persons who identify themselves with the hearing world. She acknowledges that the gap is fearful because it identifies an abyss into which one is jettisoned alone. And it appears that while in there, one is destined to remain alone. But as Sandra slowly learnt, one is not alone. Sandra stumbled her way through the process of being Deafened, endured the battle and found places where her difference was accepted and the sense of deficit to some extent, was extinguished.

At the same time, Sandra worked to maintain her connectedness with the hearing world, particularly with her children, for whom she has endured most. Sandra has found a way to achieve a sameness that does not completely disrupt her attachments with the hearing world. The sense of deficit created by the biomechanical model of the body is extinguished by engaging in a process of constantly reworking relations that produce sameness, where sameness is understood as a sense of coherency, as an experience of the continuity of self and a connectedness with others:

> 'Sameness' is a quality of our relation to the world, our assimilation of it, our interaction with it, and our appropriation of it. 'Sameness' is a cognitive stance that we take toward existence, a stance that is replicated and reinforced through its functioning in willing. In this case, identity is never closed or exclusive; it is never metaphysically guaranteed because it constantly must be constructed and reconstructed. (Warren, 1988: 201)

Sameness is achieved because life goes on. Sameness is produced by constant change. The issue of sameness is about finding a way to get on with things, of building new networks of people and re-establishing old ones, even if one's overall life experience has been marginalized. Sandra's life history demonstrates that the system of governance generally imposed upon and accepted by Deafened adults is not all encompassing. Sandra has carved out a place for herself in differing worlds. It is a compromise, the least worst outcome that enabled her to identify with Deaf people, and to maintain contact with her family. Sandra also considered a cochlear implant but rejected it because the benefits of implantation (as they were at that time) did not outweigh, in her mind, what it involved. She was advised that she would still have to lip-read and would not be able to use the telephone in all but limited circumstances. She would still be too deaf to be a hearing person and she now found enjoyment and acceptance living as a Deafened person. Most Deafened people do not appear to arrive at this point of identity integration, either prior to or after their involvement with hearing services.

Jan

Jan, as we have seen, suddenly acquired hearing loss when she was in her early teens. Fitted with high-powered hearing aids and placed within a mainstream school, Jan's experience of surviving school followed Sandra's. After completing initial post-school training, Jan held down a number of jobs before being laid off at age 21, as a result of an occupational health injury. It was about this time that Jan joined a support group for young Deafened adults and a process of transition began. She became quite active within the group and took on organizational responsibilities. But Jan did not find the group satisfying, particularly because it met infrequently, leaving her with many unfilled hours each day. Bored with her life, she left and became involved with a voluntary service organizing services for Deaf people. Here, Jan was surrounded by signing Deaf people and she began to sign herself. During this time, Jan also got a cochlear implant and became involved in providing peer support for other cochlear implantees.

Like Sandra, Jan stresses the importance of having access to people who have 'walked the talk', that is, people who have been through the process of having gone deaf and of having to select new ways to communicate and sustain a positive life. Jan identifies other people, who unlike herself, have not moved over or who are very much caught in a borderland between Deaf and hearing worlds, who continue to judge themselves against an ableist model of what being a hearing person might mean and in doing so, finding themselves lacking, in debt as it were (Disprose, 1993), to hearing society.

Jan's experience of deafness and family life reveals a process of emotional and social *divestment* that is coupled with an emergent identity as a Deafened person. For Jan, her deafness, the most structuring aspect of her life, could not be discussed at home:

> [My deafness] was just never talked about. I don't really know what they feel because we've [never] sat down and talked about it. And it was funny. I made the observation, I turned twenty-six last year and I realized that at that stage that I had spent exactly half of my life hearing and half of my life deaf! Now that sounds weird doesn't it! Yeah. And I told that to my mum ... and you should have seen her she was so ... how do you put it, shocked. She'd never thought about it. But she immediately switched herself off. So I don't think I've ever really thought about it.

Starr (1991) suggests that the experience of multiple selves serves as a critical point of analysis for understanding the taken-for-grantedness of everyday interactions and the so-called stability of social practices which are in fact quite unstable for many people. For Deafened people, it is the very taken-for-granted experience of communicating verbally on a daily basis that creates an experience of marginality. For Deafened people the hearing world 'is distinctly not ordered. Rather, it is a source of chaos and trouble' (Starr, 1991: 42).

Jan developed friendships with Deaf and Deafened people who were involved in the various movements she had joined. Jan's emotional stake in home is still high – these people are family. But like Sandra, Jan draws emotional satisfaction from her new network, while retaining an attachment to the old. Jan describes this network as a solid group of people on whom she can rely for support and understanding. For Jan it is also a two-way street, for she clearly gives a lot of support to people as well:

> The benefit of being with Deaf people is that in some ways we've still got the same problems with hearing people. I mean if we're speaking with someone and you can't understand something and you ask them to repeat it, you're not treated as if you're stupid or that you have no IQ or you have absolutely nothing between your ears except cotton wool, which often happens with hearing people. Hearing people just cannot seem to understand that it is a communication problem. The fact that I have a full brain of brain cells and they are all working is not relevant. It's simply because it could be anything. Umm someone could have walked between us or all of a sudden some background noise could have started up or they went like this ... and covered their mouth or it could be anything, they could have turned away or they could have said a word I may not have caught. All of that does not occur to hearing people at all. With Deaf people, you are generally accepted for what you are. And I've got a

> strong network of Deaf people that I can count on for support. Um, I am friends with and go out and rage. Umm, or simply just talk to. Some are implantees. Some are mildly hearing-impaired. Some are full deaf, some are in between. It's just a mixed bag.

Jan describes herself as a person with two passports, one into the hearing world and one into the deaf world. Her communication skills enable her to move between the two. Each world brings with it benefits and hassles:

> I could not spend all of my time in either world. I just could not pick one or the other. So when I get sick of hearing people um I go and mix with Deaf people and when I've had enough of Deaf people, I go and mix with hearing people. So I consider myself lucky and privileged that I am accepted in both.

Concluding remarks

Sandra and Jan's life histories problematize the classical notions of Deaf and Hearing worlds. Although their lives appear to be quite different, Sandra and Jan's worlds are both Deaf and Hearing, never being entirely one or the other. They have moved beyond the commonsense world of oralism to take up aspects of Deaf culture while retaining distinctive oral traits such as lip-reading, the cochlear implant, flashing lights, hearing dogs, hearing and speech. The activity of moving between worlds, is significant. *Moving over* is an ongoing, active process where individuals construct themselves in response to the communication environments encountered. As Warren (1988) points out, agency enables the individual to differentiate between practices which benefit as distinct from those which disadvantage. Thus the process of equipping oneself for communication is about fabricating one's identity; of actively shaping how one is to be seen by society when this presentation of self may envelope multiple forms supported by a diversity of technologies. The nature of identity depends on where one is, with whom and what one is doing at the time.

There are many ways to live out being deafened. The process of decision-making associated with being deafened is influenced by what Moore (1994) identifies as the extent of one's personal investment in particular people or associations. Similarly, Dowsett (1994: 67-71) develops the notion of attachment when discussing identification with the Gay community:

> attachment is not something a person possesses to a greater or lesser degree, but a process of constructing a meaningful daily life within a collectively produced social frame ... there is no single community; there are only ever-changing dominant cultural forms and identities supported, in some cases, by an increasingly sophisticated urban infrastructure. (p. 71)

Sandra and Jan gradually developed personal investments in diverse networks over long periods of time. Carol did not. It is evident then that there is a point to work to, or to avoid, in which a process of personal formation may result in the development of a disability identity that incorporates into one's lifestyle and networks the acceptance or rejection of specific discursive practices. Some people, such as Sandra and Jan, are able to take on specific practices, and involve themselves in new networks wherein they may (or may not) be identified as Deaf, as disabled, as other. If the onset of deafness symbolizes a chasm, a deafness identity symbolizes a light at the end of the tunnel. Central to developing this new identity is the recognition, by Deafened people and others, of the experience of heterogeneity that deafness creates; an experience that is not necessarily negative. As Starr (1991) observes:

> Multiple marginality is a source not only of monstrosity and impurity, but of a power that at once resists violence and encompasses heterogeneity. (p. 30)

Present clinical practices allow little opportunity for Deafened people to recognize or to work through their experience of multiple selves, contested identity or their multiple encounters with marginality. Clinics work from the assumption that Deafened people are only marginalized from Hearing culture and that there is an understandable legitimacy in such marginality. From the clinic's perspective, the solution is to assimilate Deafened people back into Hearing culture. Rehabilitation providers need to examine the presumption that simply because people are deaf, they would want to be 'just' hearing people, or that a technology-based intervention (such as the cochlear implant) is necessarily the intervention of 'first choice' or only choice.

Rather the first point of intervention may be an encounter between the newly Deafened people and their networks, with people such as Sandra and Jan, coupled with a facilitated introduction to the politics of disability, practice and personal identity. Once clients and those close to them have had the opportunity to work through their fears about disability and discrimination and to develop the necessary assertiveness and communication skills they require, they will be much better equipped to make the most of what advanced technologies such as cochlear implants can offer. This is the model underpinning the Link Centre for Deafened Adults in Eastbourne (United Kingdom). This programme is able to improve a person's quality of life substantially with a one-week intensive rehabilitation and socializing experience. It clearly has a lot going for it.

Summary

Deafened adults report having a reduced quality of life, high unemployment and under employment and mostly live on low incomes. The onset of deafness results in an experience of contested identity. Contested identity, coupled with a marginalized social position and problematized social interactions have physical and emotional consequences in addition to the social problems experienced. When Deafened people present at the clinic for assistance, they are not simply seeking resolution of their hearing difficulties, but relief from the overall problems that deafness brought into their lives. In such circumstances, clinicians are faced with the challenge of engaging people into a change and an affirmation process – not simply an assessment and device fitting procedure. Figure 1.6 provides an overview of the rehabilitation process. It provides a map of the rehabilitation pathway that lies ahead.

Many of the issues that have been addressed so far in this text provide the background that in turn will inform and make coherent the rehabilitation strategies provided in Part II. Not least of these is the recognition of the marginal social status of Deafened adults and therefore why it is necessary to actively recruit Deafened adults into the healing process. The continuing focus of this text addresses the needs of Deafened adults likely to benefit from a cochlear implant. Indeed, a variety of barriers exist that prevent this group easily reaching the clinic. Elsewhere, Louise Getty and Raymond Hetu (1991) have detailed strategies for recruiting other Deafened people into the rehabilitation process. Specifically, this involves a recruitment strategy using a trusted person as the link between the client and the clinic. Time and again, I have found their strategy to be relevant and indicated, not just with people with mild to moderate losses, but for the more severely deafened as well.

The social position of Deafened people means that there are factors that predispose people not to seek help and/or reinforce (i.e. validate) inaction. When caught up in passing and compliant behaviours, one's focus is centred on fitting in and not dealing with the interpersonal consequences of one's deafness. Indeed, to address deafness is to make visible that which stigmatizes. A transition process, like a rite of passage, is therefore required in order to commence a change process. An active recruitment strategy is the first step in helping to commence this problem-solving endeavour.

Part II
Addressing Psychosocial Issues within Rehabilitation Programmes for Deafened People

Chapter 4

Addressing everyday barriers to cochlear implantation

Preamble

In Part II the focus of this text moves from the theoretical to the practical. While not forgetting the broader social issues that impact on the Deafened person and the adjustment process, attention now focuses on addressing the needs identified. The benefits of cochlear implantation are such that to my mind, they form a central, but not a total part of the rehabilitation process. The cochlear implant addresses, to an extent, sensory loss. While such benefits are generally extensive, they are also varied. While many people, particularly in recent times, gain an enormous auditory benefit from the device, their psychosocial and family issues must also be addressed. Taken together, and not excluding the use of signing, a powerful arsenal of assistance is now available to the Deafened adult. Within civilized societies, appropriate efforts need to be made to ensure that these interventions reach those who benefit from them.

This chapter examines issues that may prevent a Deafened person from gaining ready access to an implant programme. First, attention is given to attitudes Deafened adults may hold towards cochlear implants. Second, attitudes of private and community-based audiologists to cochlear implants are also considered. Based on the evidence reported, strategies for enhancing client access to the programme are discussed. A tension exists here with regard to how the Deafened person is defined – as patient, client, etc. Following the social model of disability, I shall use the term client.

Deafened adults generally acquired their profound loss of hearing between the ages of 35 to 50 years. An adjustment period of some years followed before people were prepared to seek implantation, although this factor is now beginning to change as the management of profound deafness moves from a chronic to acute models of care. Following the onset of loss, Deafened people have a number of personal and social issues to work through prior to considering something as significant as a cochlear implant. They utilize a variety of rehabilitation services, indicating a preparedness to 'shop around' for rehabilitation outcomes. Conversely, audiologists' behaviour was strongly influenced by the extent to which they had knowledge about the implant programme and had some degree of contact with it.

Awareness of, knowledge concerning, and confidence in, the cochlear implant were also identified as key factors inhibiting prospective candidates from seeking implantation. The provision of information and support services targeting both audiologists and prospective clients, coupled with a slightly diversified rehabilitation intervention, may greatly enhance referrals made to a specific implant clinic.

Introduction

Despite the ready availability of cochlear implant technology and the absence of significant client-incurred costs necessarily associated with the procedure (implants may be publicly and/or insurer funded in many western countries), comparatively few potentially eligible adults have been implanted to date. In Australia for example, only some 500 adults have been implanted to date and there are some 28,000 Deafened and non-signing adults who may potentially benefit from the technology. This low take-up rate suggests the possibility that barriers may exist that prevent Deafened adults from accessing the implant programme. This chapter reports on a study concerned to identify what barriers, if any, impact upon client decision-making processes associated with cochlear implantation.

Managing your referral sources

Deafened adults primarily see a small number of professionals concerning their hearing loss. These are their general practitioner (53%), their audiologists (100%) and ear, nose and throat specialists (73%). Efforts to recruit implant candidates should therefore be targeted primarily at these bodies. Presently, there is little data available on the attitudes of doctors concerning cochlear implants, although preliminary work has shown that only 13 per cent of GPs had referred a client to an implant clinic. However, recent data has been collected on the attitudes and referral behaviours of audiologists working outside the implant programme. This research shows that the readiness of a specific audiologist to refer a potential candidate to an implant clinic is influenced by the following factors:

1. their experience with previous implant clients;
2. preparedness to discuss implants with clients;
3. existence of a working relationship between the audiologist and an implant clinic;
4. knowledge as to how to make an effective referral for implantation;
5. where the audiologist was employed;
6. satisfaction with the nature and extent of training they had received on implants;
7. awareness of funding options for new implant clients;
8. confidence in the rehabilitation process to produce a satisfactory client outcome.

Most audiologists are aware of cochlear implants and have a good working knowledge of what the device can offer a client. Nonetheless, candidates have received mixed advice from professionals working in the field about the technology, most specifically, that they were either unsuitable for implantation (when they actually were) or that they should wait until the technology is perfected.

About two-thirds (65%) of audiologists studied had in fact referred a client to an implant clinic for an assessment. Audiologists who were less likely to refer a prospective candidate indicated either:

1. a desire for more training on implants;
2. were less experienced; and/or
3. lived outside the metropolitan area.

It is important therefore, to ensure that audiologists and general practitioners working in your catchment area, especially new graduates:

1. are up-to-date on what the implant can offer clients;
2. are aware of the referral criteria;
3. are familiar with the procedure for initiating a referral;
4. understand the follow-up mechanisms for keeping in contact with you;
5. are familiar with issues to assist country people access to your clinic with ease;
6. understand funding options (public and private) available to prospective clients;
7. are aware of the process for updating speech processes;
8. are aware of the capacity of surgeons to implant new electrode designs should this be indicated.

Most audiologists see someone who might be eligible for an implant occasionally. However, most audiologists have limited exposure to implantees with 75 per cent having never worked with more than five implantees. Interestingly, those audiologists who had referred people for implants exhibited a positive working relationship with their local implant centre. They thought implants were effective, safe and reliable. In particular, experienced audiologists expressed satisfaction with the progress of implantees. Nonetheless, these audiologists remained unclear about the correct referral criteria for severely hearing-impaired clients and wanted more information on how to manage the psychological support needs of prospective candidates.

It is evident then that those professionals most likely to refer a client for an implant assessment have specific and ongoing information needs. Regular orientation and open days at your implant clinic may facilitate communication with these professionals, therein resulting in a smoother transition for the Deafened client to the clinic. It needs to be kept in mind that while audiologists generally have a positive attitude towards cochlear implants and have an adequate level of device knowledge, they are unlikely to refer candidates for an implant unless they know their local implant provider and are confident that their client will receive the type of intervention they require.

Who is the prospective implant client?

People presenting for implants are likely to have been Deafened relatively early in life and during their working years. The mean age of deafness onset for current implantees is approximately age 40 (s.d. 18 years). Of those implantees Deafened in the last five years, 56 per cent were aged less than 60 years. For those Deafened post-1986, the mean duration of deafness prior to implantation was four years (s.d. 3 years). For those Deafened in the last five years, the mean duration of deafness prior to implantation was 1.7 years (s.d. 1.7 years). Seventy-five per cent of all people implanted in the last five years had been Deafened for more than six years, with 49 per cent having been deaf for more than 15 years. These data show that while recently Deafened people may move quite efficiently into the implant system, the majority of people presenting have been deaf for a long time and have quite specific management needs. Nonetheless, the onset of deafness presents the client with an additional mid-life crisis to contend with, particularly given that this is a key period in any person's work and family life.

There are a number of factors that may motivate a person with long-term deafness to present for further assistance. These factors include:

1. becoming aware of the technology (or their eligibility for it) for the first time;
2. progressive loss of remaining hearing;
3. change in personal circumstances (e.g. relationship pressures).

It needs to be kept in mind that this person has lived successfully as a Deafened adult for a long time. Something significant has happened to bring them at this stage to present for a cochlear implant. This factor needs to be explored during the initial interview (see Chapter 6).

Attitudes to implants

One of the social consequences of hearing loss is reduced employment opportunities and in turn, lower incomes. The cost of the implant is therefore an issue for prospective clients, particularly those who cannot afford private health insurance and in countries where there is no (or limited) publicly funded implants. A second issue is the nature of the speech processor, many of which are cumbersome to manage. To an extent this problem has been greatly overcome with the development of the ear-level processor, but then such processors are limited by problems with power supply and/or the type of information they can carry. Nonetheless, there are times and places where the device cannot be used effectively, such as swimming. The enduring concern for clinicians and potential implantees is the fact that implant technology, irrespective of the manufacturer concerned, is constantly being changed. It certainly is a useful technology but, from a consumer perspective, it is far from being perfect as individuals confront nagging problems on a day-to-day basis. These concerns (like telephone access) should not be discounted with comments such as 'well it is much better than nothing at all'. Daily frustrations require acknowledgement and support.

One of the key issues concerning Deafened adults is the idea that they will either lose their capacity to lip-read or that they will still need to lip-read, following implantation. This information needs to be managed carefully. What appears to happen post-implant is that a client's reliance on visual clues is greatly reduced. It would be true to say that many implantees will still need to lip-read; however, the level of effort entailed is greatly reduced, due to the increased auditory benefit they now enjoy. It is not that the skill is lost as much as the client is utilizing the benefits that the technology can offer. Additional concerns reflect client perceptions that the sound of the device will be insufficient or unusable, and that telephone access will not be achieved. Recall in Part I where we discussed the fact that clients want their lives back, to have things as they once were.

Put another way, they want to restore the quality of life that they have lost. The evidence is now available which shows that for the majority of clients, implantation results in a significantly enhanced quality of life and reduction in day-to-day communication difficulties. Information concerning changes in the use of skills like lip-reading then need to be discussed in the context of how the rehabilitation intervention will, as a whole, enable them to *get back on with their lives*.

As the implant programme moves from a chronic model of care (managing those who have been deaf for a long time) to an acute model of care (where the client is the newly Deafened adult), rehabilitation and access services will need to take into account the socio-economic issues that impact upon them. Many new prospective implantees are of working age and may, as a result of their newly acquired deafness, be at risk of losing their employment or have lost considerable income as a result of unemployment. The provision of assessments and rehabilitation services during extended hours, perhaps in a similar fashion to those offered in dentistry, may greatly assist clients during a difficult time of adjustment.

Despite the fact that various cochlear implants have received safety approval from bodies such as the American Food and Drug administration, client perceptions of implant safety remain an issue. The key issues concerning safety are the potential loss of their residual hearing (i.e. leave them worse off than they are now) and the short- as well as longer-term possible effects of implantation. These are factors that also need to be addressed during pre-implant counselling.

Awareness of eligibility for an implant

Interviews with implantees and prospective candidates indicate that client awareness about the device is low and is primarily accessed through media portrayals of the device, especially in community newspapers and resourceful friends. Small numbers of candidates sought out a referral for implantation, based upon their own knowledge about the availability of the technology, gleaned from access to academic journals and the general media. Certainly, a candidate's decision to seek out implantation is swayed both by the information offered and the manner in which it is delivered. Some health professionals adopt a *wait and see approach* while others actively seek to shape the client's decision. Health professionals not in favour of an implant can have both positive and negative effects. On the one hand, by adopting the role of advocate/service broker, health professionals can ensure that the prospective candidate is aware of all their options. In one instance, a health provider tried to prevent a candidate from proceeding to seek out implantation by providing the person with a range of 'anti-implant' materials. The net effect was that if the so-called 'worst' was in fact the worst that could happen, then it was worth the risk in the person's own mind.

The provision of information about what is really likely to happen in and/or following implantation is pivotal to the decision-making process. The client's reluctance to seek out an assessment was overcome by realistic information about the implant process. On the other hand, a client's reluctance may also be intensified by the way information is provided and the manner in which it is delivered. Reluctance is a complex psychological phenomenon that receives further attention in the next chapter.

Deafened adults considering implantation require access to accurate, timely, and 'balanced' information about the nature and reliability of the cochlear implant. Access to such information could be greatly enhanced by the provision of education materials targeted at the general community, including directions on acquiring further information where needed.

Awareness of the suitability of a particular Deafened person for an implant remains an issue. Many people believe that implants are only for 'totally' deaf people, with this perception being high among those who have discussed implantation with their doctor or audiologist. The problem with referring agents is not that they will not refer, rather that they do not refer. The barrier here being with people who have longer standing deafness and who, in consequence, are managed as people with a chronic rather than an acute condition, where the need for referral or for further consideration of impairment management is not so apparent. This barrier is further complicated by the fact that many people are getting on with their lives as Deafened adults, and consider that they are doing fine without the technology. While this may well be true for some, the data show that this group in fact experiences a significantly reduced quality of life (Hogan et al., 2000). 'Getting on fine' may in fact refer to the person making the most of the situation they find themselves in, not wanting to complain and so on, rather than being a statement that reflects them having optimized their life opportunities. Indeed, approximately one-third of Deafened people surveyed reported dissatisfaction with both the services they had received and the outcomes achieved (Hogan, 1996).

Summary

Following the onset of advanced hearing impairment, Deafened adults work to stabilize their lives. For most, this stabilization consists of a steady process of adaptation over long periods of time. Rarely have such individuals encountered a cochlear implant programme. Awareness of implant centres results from luck (e.g. media) or through coming to know someone with an implant, perhaps through a self-help group. There is no clear pathway that guides people to the conclusion that they might consider having a cochlear implant. Longer term Deafened adults, including the severely hearing-impaired, require access to a check list that informs them when it is time to seek advice about cochlear implants. By contrast, those suddenly Deafened find themselves more able to engage implant clinics and give consideration to the use of the technology simply because they used hospital-based services.

Discussion

Barriers to cochlear implantation can be summarized as awareness, knowledge and confidence. The inaccessibility of cochlear implant referral, information and assessment processes is underscored by an absence of information and access skills amongst potential service users. Awareness barriers have two aspects. First, Deafened people are not simply unaware of implant centres, they are unaware of their eligibility for an implant in clinical as well as financial terms. Second, they are unaware as to what they can do to redress their deafness generally. Once aware, they need confidence and support to negotiate the process. This barrier appears to be addressed by the availability of (often voluntary) rehabilitation advocates. As such a rehabilitation advocates' programme is indicated. The role of such advocates would be to:

1. act as a link between audiology clinics and other potential referral centres (e.g. self-help groups, employment services) and implant clinics;
2. assist prospective candidates to access appropriate information so that they may make informed decisions about their rehabilitation programme (including the viability, safety and suitability of an implant given their particular circumstances);
3. assist prospective candidates to negotiate their rehabilitation programme in conjunction with their employer, insurer, health service purchaser/provider or similar body.

Lack of access to reliable information concerning cochlear implantation means that potential candidates do not seek out a referral for implantation. This reluctance stems, in part, from concerns about possible injury. Such community concern may have been fuelled by the anti-cochlear implant campaign mounted by the Deaf community in earlier times. In consequence, objective data concerning the safety and reliability of the device needs to be more readily available to prospective candidates. To this end it is incumbent on clinics to make data available to clients on the following issues:

- The market status of the technology on offer – is it current? Is it likely to be superseded in the near future? How does it compare with other devices on the market (what is the basis of this comparison)? It is safe and reliable – if so, to what extent as compared with alternative devices?
- The nature of diagnostics used in the clinic, their accuracy and usefulness, information about less invasive alternatives that may be available at other clinics, particularly those in the same city.
- The likelihood of benefits arising from (1) the surgery and subsequent rehabilitation; (2) other forms of aural rehabilitation available or that could be provided.
- Factors unique to the clients' situation that may impact adversely on the likely outcome.
- Information on complementary and alternative therapies.

User perspectives

Current paradigms for reporting scientific research, provide little room for subjective perspectives of the people who actually get implanted. However, from a clinical perspective, the views of Deafened people concerning their experiences of implantation are critical. There have been some 'scary' stories about the terrors of cochlear implantation promoted by people who are against the device. Invariably, prospective candidates come to know of such stories – so they need to be dealt with in a positive and informative manner.

Client motivation to pursue implant technology

Like many people with an acquired illness or disability, Deafened people have waited for science to develop a cure for their hearing loss. The heralded arrival of the implant signalled to Deafened people a dream come true. Deafened people sought out an implant because they wanted to be part of the hearing world – they wanted to hear and speak. It is not that Deafened people necessarily reject the world of signing Deaf people, it is simply that deafness results in an experience of marginality from which they seek to be liberated. This marginality is itself a barrier to people seeking help and often it is not that clients lack motivation, but rather that clinics lack an adequate recruitment process that serves as the major barrier to service delivery to larger numbers of people.

Risk

As most clinicians involved in the cochlear implant programme know, Deafened adults present for implantation in the hope that with the device that they will regain most, if not all of their hearing. In consequence, the preliminary work with the client is concerned with the management of these expectations. Part of this responsibility is working with the client, not just to give them a realistic expectation of their likely outcome, but to enable them to understand what is involved in the overall rehabilitation process, including the risks associated with surgery. Certainly fear of surgery or the risks associated with it, are a barrier to implantation.

Deafened people can cope with the fact that problems may be associated with implantation. Problems associated with the process are managed within a hierarchy of risks, consequences and benefits that are weighed up by the individual candidate. Reflecting on her approaching surgery, one client remarked:

> I had nothing to lose. I wanted to hear again, but mainly because I had nothing to lose. I was born hearing and any chance that would possibly give me some hearing back would be welcome.

The ability of clients to seek out and weigh up risk stands in contrast to the belief that candidates should be told as little as possible about the risks associated with surgery. The ethical issue is not so much the notion of risk, but the right to decide. And of course, it is a fundamental right that prospective candidates make an informed consent to surgery. What has concerned implantees the most has not been so much the possibility of an adverse event, but the absence of up-front information provided to them prior to surgery. Power relations between Deafened adults and implant clinics are asymmetrical. Without an advocate and in the absence of alternative sources of information, the Deafened person is reliant upon the professional's judgement and advice, viewpoints already shaped by values reflecting an understanding of the nature and meaning of impairment and the personal impact of surgery. Managing a decision-making process without power can be disabling in itself for candidates. It erodes independence and self-confidence and requires subjects to make an unnecessary deference to a professional based solely on trust. From the perspective of the implantee, the process of cochlear implantation is not necessarily straightforward; it can be traumatic and injurious. In addition, events that some surgeons may consider trivial (e.g. transient tinnitus or temporary facial palsy) may in fact be quite stressful for the implantee.

Certainly implantees do not enter the programme uninformed about the likely risks associated with the procedure. However, much can and ought to be done to improve the information process to ensure that prospective implantees have access to information about the process that is comprehensive, up-to-date, ideally provided by a third party (e.g. social work department) and within a process that is designed to ensure that likely candidates are fully aware that the technology and the surgical process associated with it are constantly being improved.

CHAPTER 5

Psychosocial approaches to hearing rehabilitation: it's a matter of process

Introduction

Following the onset of hearing loss, individuals and their partners may experience a range of adverse psychosocial consequences that are directly associated with their disability. These consequences may include increased stress, anxiety, isolation, loss of job, reduced income, loss of life partner and reduced health (Hetu and Getty, 1991; Getty and Hetu, 1991; Hogan, 1997; Wilson, 1997). Participation in rehabilitative processes (e.g. hearing aid use; cochlear implants) does not guarantee that these problems will go away. Indeed, they tend to hang around. The limitation of more traditional approaches to hearing rehabilitation has been their focus on behavioural components of rehabilitation (e.g. strategies and technologies) while the psychosocial fundamentals of adjustment to disability remain unaddressed.

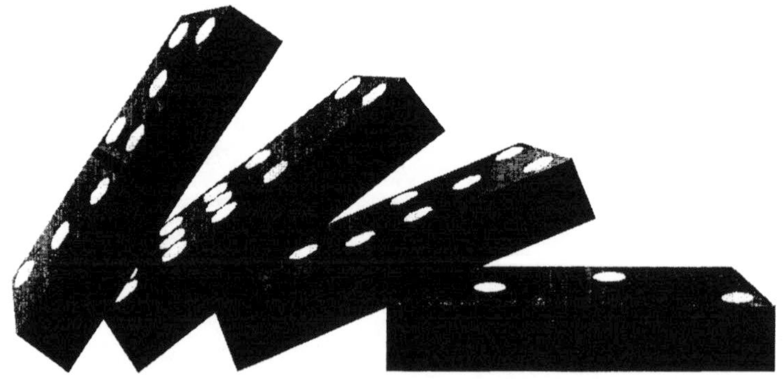

Figure 5.1: Hearing tactics have psychological consequences.

The process of adjustment to hearing disability is associated with changes in a variety of psychosocial domains including identity and belief systems. It is a process of learning to understand that, despite deafness, one is the same person while experiencing life differently.

The extent of changes achieved within psychosocial domains directly influences changes in behaviour, the development of communication competencies and the appropriate use of technologies. The process of adjustment is hampered by the dynamics of misperception and reluctance (Hetu and Getty, 1991; Getty and Hetu, 1991). The nature of misperception varies depending on the outcomes of the disability/impairment dyad. Many are familiar with the notion of misperception where people attribute hearing difficulties to factors such as not wanting to socialize, changed interests, people mumbling and so on. Reluctance on the other hand can encompass strategies where people seek to minimize the extent of their impairment or avoid using strategies that might otherwise be helpful. Experiences of *reluctance* on the part of people with hearing impairment may be understood as being part of a process whereby the individual adjusts to both the way they relate to others and the way in which they may understand themselves. The spontaneous development of coping strategies may be based on a fear of marginalization and, in fact, serve to socially isolate the deafened adult further.

Living with hearing loss entails a process of learning to be the same while being different. Within the rehabilitation process, clients work to develop a new sense of the old self, where a positive outcome entails the development of effective strategies for getting on with one's life, as near to what they had hoped for as possible, while positively integrating the types of changes necessary to living successfully with hearing loss. Central to the rehabilitation process is the need to enable the client to understand the social dynamics of communication that have so often resulted in a sense of stigmatization. Within social interactions, people with hearing loss are often left with a sense of being put down or being blameworthy when interpersonal communication fails. Through the use of communication tactics and peer education, clients come to realize that there are many things that they can do to reduce the stress of social interactions, to enhance their communication skills and to manage, in an assertive fashion, problematic communication settings (e.g. a visit to a restaurant). Left unaided, it may take more than ten years for the hearing-impaired person to work through the adjustment process and, even then, the adjustments achieved may be less than the individual might have hoped for (Hogan, 1998b). Inadequate adjustment to disability may result in such increased levels of stress that Deafened adults experience increased levels of illness and loss of quality of life.

Background to psychosocial approaches in aural rehabilitation

Hearing rehabilitation has been the focus of professional interest for centuries. Edwards (1994), for example, reports that in Ancient Greece practitioners sought to treat deafness by removing wax from the ear canal. More recent models of hearing rehabilitation began in the nineteenth century in the United Kingdom, Europe and the United States (Hogan, 1997). These forms of rehabilitation focused on the development of the Deafened person's communication skills. Following the Second World War centres were established for the rehabilitation of soldiers with hearing loss resulting from battle noise such as cannons and other explosions (Gaeth, 1979). The rehabilitation programme was a multi-disciplinary approach that consisted of learning to understand hearing loss, developing communication strategies and learning to listen with and manage amplified sound. These programmes continually emphasized working with the whole person. Gaeth remarked:

> A man is more important than his ears. Specialists in hearing and speech proceed in the belief that they are under obligation to treat the total personality. (1979: 8)

Gaeth noted that client-centred programmes focused on two key points:

1. the development of new abilities and skills, to achieve efficient and successful behaviour and adjustment;
2. the understanding and nullification of the adverse effects that are inevitable by-producers of any serious interference with communicative habits.

Programmes were offered both on an individual basis and in groups. As military personnel, the participant's job was to be in the programme.

The rubella epidemic followed on soon after the war and in countries such as Australia intensive resources were focused on the development of intensive hearing rehabilitation programmes for children (Cordell, 1978). In consequence, the urgent need to provide large numbers of children with a comprehensive hearing rehabilitation programme meant that holistic approaches to adult hearing rehabilitation fell away – the adult programme became almost exclusively technology focused. Although the rubella epidemic is now long past, there has been no systematic catalyst that has served to refocus institutions to the need that adults also require a dynamic model of rehabilitation.

Despite these institutional limitations, various hearing rehabilitation providers have worked to develop a range of models that offer what might be called a ***psychosocial approach*** to hearing rehabilitation. The psychosocial approach to hearing rehabilitation has several key aims. These are to:

1. improve the participants' general quality of life, including that of significant others;
2. reduce the extent of hearing disability (or what is sometimes referred to as hearing handicap) experienced by the participants and their partners through the development of appropriate knowledge, self-confidence and communication skills;
3 ensure that the participants and their partners have access to the types of hearing technologies most appropriate to their communication needs;
4. look at cost-effective methods for delivering these services.

Various hearing rehabilitation providers have been offering psychosocial approaches in hearing rehabilitation for more than twenty years (Pengilley, 1975; Plant, 1976; Plant, 1977; Hetu and Getty, 1991; Getty and Hetu, 1991; Hogan et al., 1994; Anderson, 1991; Sherbourne and White, 1997; Westcott and Kato, 1998). Key features of these interventions have been:

1. group-based interventions;
2. the involvement of people with hearing impairment and their spouses or close friends (the spouses were involved in the process because 'they themselves bear the effects of the reduced listening and communication abilities of their husbands ... the spouses are likely to react positively to an offer of professional help ... the spouses do not understand the nature of the impairments, their spontaneous reactions to communication difficulties are very often a source of handicap for the worker ... [and since] the major effects of OHL appear to be experienced in the family' (Getty and Hetu: 1991: 45);
3. a multi-disciplinary team approach, often including peer educators;
4. a process model of peer education where the focus of the programme centres on the lived experience of hearing-impaired people dealing with problematic communication settings;
5. outcomes evaluation – these programmes have demonstrated measurable improvements in participants' quality of life and reductions in hearing disability.

Central to the successful implementation of these programmes has been the combination of the materials used and the style of presentation.

Commonly, such interventions are offered either intensively over several days or programmatically over several weeks. The style of intervention centres on group-based problem-solving and topics centre upon resolving problematized communication settings.

The idea that hearing rehabilitation extends beyond the realm of fitting a hearing aid or other technology is not new. Plant (1976: 15-19) notes that the Australian Government's National Acoustic Laboratory has long recognized 'that the mere fitting of a hearing aid is not a satisfactory solution to the many problems confronting the adventitiously deaf'. Plant argued that follow-up programmes in groups and for individuals which are concerned with hearing aid orientation, hearing tactics and speech-reading classes are necessary. He particularly notes the need of extra support for people with mild to moderate hearing losses. Plant points out that 'the audiologist conducting the programme attempts to become a group leader rather than a lecturer'. The programme aims to give people 'a realistic attitude' towards managing their difficulties. Plant also notes the success of Scandinavian hearing rehabilitation programmes that are offered along similar lines. Currently, the Australian Hearing Services offers seriously deafened adults intensive communication training and support via residential workshops (Westcott and Kato, 1998). Participants in cochlear implant programmes are also beginning to take part in group-based interventions (Hogan, 1998b).

Perhaps one of the better known and documented approaches to psychosocial rehabilitation is the programme developed by Louise Getty and Raymond Hetu (English translation by Anthony Hogan, 1992). This French-Canadian model centres on a process of facilitated, group-based, problem-solving where people with acquired hearing loss and their spouses develop communication skills and attitudes appropriate to their hearing rehabilitation needs. Central to the successful implementation of this programme was the provider's capacity to engage participants in a problem-solving process wherein the service user is enabled to identify and understand problems caused by their hearing impairment and to investigate solutions which they may consider relevant to their needs. During this problem-solving process, participants are introduced to topics such as understanding the ear, stress management, hearing tactics, complementary therapies, hearing aids and assistive listening devices. The Link Centre's service (Eastbourne, United Kingdom) offers a similar intervention to severely and profoundly Deafened adults.

The psychosocial model is then:

1. a process model of rehabilitation;
   - that pivots on interactions and experiences of group members
   - that occurs within a semi-structured setting;

2. facilitated by hearing rehabilitation professionals and/or peer educators;
3. seeking to develop confidence and assertiveness in clients.

This method of intervention is quite similar to a model of social research known as action research. Within action research, participants and providers work on equal footing to identify and work through problems of interest (Mergler, 1987). There is no core regime of treatment per se; instead communication problems and barriers arise and are resolved with a problem-solving process centred on discussions, group-work and peer interactions. This process is pedagogically different to individualizing device-centred models of intervention because at the end of the day hearing is about communication and communication is a social process.

Contrasting approaches

Group-based interventions then are distinctly different to hearing rehabilitation programmes focused almost exclusively on the provision of technologies.

First, the intervention is centred on a problem-solving process that people engage in – the rehabilitation process is centred on and driven by the participants themselves. The stories people tell are the foundational materials upon which the remainder of the intervention pivots. Technology-centred services inherently focus attempts to manage the vast array of social difficulties experienced by people with hearing loss on the strategic use of the device of interest.

Second, technology-based approaches are centred on medically styled interventions that are not entirely appropriate to the client's needs, particularly in the early stages of the rehabilitation process. Medically styled interventions concern themselves with remediating a *deficit* that has been identified within the body. Communication breakdown occurs outside the body – between bodies in fact!

The third point of variation centres on the locus of decision-making. Psychosocial interventions support participants in developing their own problem-solving assessment and decision-making skills, whereas technology-based interventions rely on the professionals to assess disability status and prescribe treatment. Most distinctly, providers of psychosocial models of rehabilitation have an arm's length arrangement with technology dispensers. For no matter how professional and objective a provider of technology may be, a prospective client rightly expects a technology provider to have an opinion as to what is the best device or collection of devices available to suit their needs. This is why one consults a provider. When a client has already undergone an appropriately structured psychosocial intervention, they are equipped to engage professionals in a decision-making process as informed and empowered consumers.

Fourth, psychosocial approaches do not undermine the benefit of hearing aids or cochlear implants as a choice a client may utilize in the rehabilitation process. Rather, it simply does not assume that technology serves as the cornerstone to successful rehabilitation. Providers of psychosocial interventions are holistic in their approach to rehabilitation since they are concerned with the whole life experience of the client, including the need for technologies and assistive devices where appropriate.

Psychosocial interventions: identifying programme goals, strategies and outcomes

Now that the nature of psychosocial approaches to hearing rehabilitation has been outlined, it is appropriate to define what a comprehensive hearing rehabilitation programme entails and seeks to achieve. This definition is important since many services function in the absence of clearly defined goals, uncertain as to what they seek to achieve beyond giving their clients some experience of sound. Within a comprehensive approach to hearing rehabilitation programmes, psychosocial and technology-based approaches (such as hearing aids, tactile devices and cochlear implants) form integral programme components.

Programme aim

A comprehensive hearing rehabilitation programme aims to improve quality of life and to reduce the experience of disability experienced by clients (deafened adults and their partners).

Programme objectives

Programme objectives may be outlined within two parallel streams, the technological and the psychosocial. Of course, the delineation is somewhat artificial, but is offered for the purposes of clarity, programme planning and evaluation. In practice, these various components may be offered interactively and/or conjointly, by a multi-disciplinary rehabilitation team.

The programme seeks to:

- enhance hearing sensitivity and reduce hearing impairment by providing participants with access to auditory stimulation appropriate to their communication needs;

- enhance participants' ability to detect speech and environmental sounds;
- enhance participants' hearing and listening skills;
- improve participants' physical health by reducing the physical/psychological demands of deafness on the body;
- reduce the extent of hearing handicap/disability experienced by participants;
- improve the partner's physical health by reducing the physical/psychological demands of deafness on the body;
- reduce the extent of shared disability experienced by partners;
- enhance the participants' socio-economic position by referring clients (on a needs basis) to appropriate employment and/or other social services.

Comprehensive hearing rehabilitation programmes employ a multidisciplinary team of professionals and peer educators, who work in close collaboration with the clients during the rehabilitation programme.

Programme structure and process: a process of facilitated self-help

As already noted, the psychosocial aspects of a hearing rehabilitation programme centre on a group-based intervention where group leaders (who are often hearing-impaired themselves) facilitate a group problem-solving interaction centred on a series of objectives such as understanding technical devices, sharing common experiences of living with hearing loss and the development of specific communication skills. A large part of each workshop within the programme is concerned with enabling clients to define, explore and resolve problematic interactional problems (Hogan et al., 1994). This is why the rehabilitation programme is referred to as a psychosocial process, rather than a course (Hetu and Getty, 1991). In this section, a description of the rehabilitation programme is given, with process notes on the purpose and application of various exercises.

The problem-solving process has specific objectives. These are:

1. to offer psychosocial support to enable clients to better deal with the effects of the hearing loss;
2. to allow the clients to understand the nature and the consequences of the problems they experience;
3. to enable clients to develop skills and attitudes that will facilitate enhanced communication outcomes (Getty and Hetu, 1991).

Programme objectives are achieved through the use of specific exercises. These exercises aim to enable participants to:

1. recognize the problems they are experiencing;
2. understand the nature and impact of these difficulties;
3. develop competencies (skills, knowledge and attitudes) to manage these.

As will become apparent as we work our way through the various exercises, different teaching materials can be used at different times during the programme, however experience has shown that some work in particular sessions better than others. The programme is implemented in a transitional fashion, commencing with exercises concerned with problem identification. In the first instance, the main aim is to get issues acknowledged and 'on the table' as it were. No attempt is made to resolve these issues. This is done in order to maintain the openness of the group experience (as problem resolution may be seen to be judgemental), but also because it takes several exercises before the full range of experiences becomes apparent. It just takes some people longer than others to open up and allowances need to be made for this very basic group dynamic. Figure 5.2 provides an overview of the programme structure.

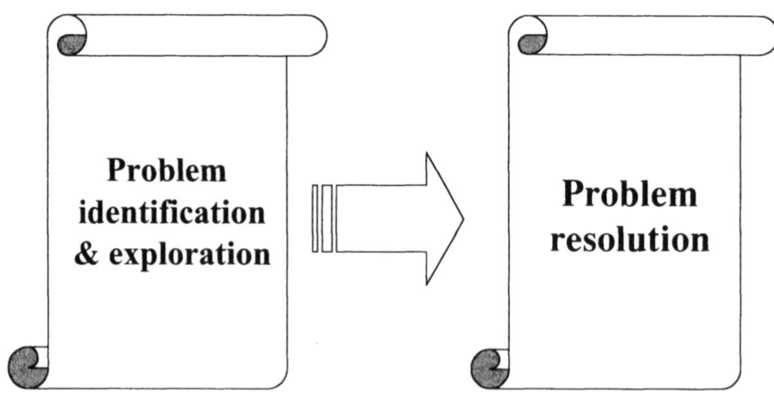

Figure 5.2: Overview.

Developing communication skills

Initially the programme focuses on *problem identification*.

The programme proper begins with participants (including spouses) taking the opportunity to acknowledge and identify the difficulties caused by their hearing impairment. The first exercise is entitled *'What's the worst thing about living with hearing loss?'* Figure 5.3 highlights the goals of this exercise. Participants are asked to answer this question in turn, beginning with the deafened participants first and then returning to partners. Support is given to participants as they describe the difficulties they experience. Since not all participants or spouses can readily express these difficulties, the group process provides a vehicle for the group leader to assist such participants to compare and contrast their experiences with those of the more articulate group members. The group leader draws upon a series of open-ended questions to enable less articulate participants to express themselves. Often, for example, a participant might simply say, 'Oh, I'm just like the other people here.' It is important, therefore, to help such people express themselves more clearly by asking questions or offering statements like:

- Well, John said he had problems talking to people at the bus stop. Can you tell me about a time when you recently had difficulties speaking with someone?
- Tell me more about that ... What's it like for you when that happens? (e.g. a person says they have a specific problem, but gives no details)
- Would you say your experience was the same as John's, is it more intensive or not as bad?
- The key difficulties likely to be reported can be seen in Figure 5.4.

What's the worst thing about living with hearing loss?

Goals

- list experiences of incongruence;
- recognize challenge to personal continuity;
- evidence role break down.

Figure 5.3: Problem identification.

- can't participate easily in conversations;
- need lots of cues and repeats;
- need key words written down;
- nerves impact on communication;
- don't use device/aid well;
- can't tell people about the problem;
- unable to ask people to help out.

Figure 5.4: Key difficulties.

Every group is different, so be open to what people have to say. While the group leader facilitates the discussion and writes notes on the whiteboard concerning people's experiences, the co-leader makes mental as well as subtle written notes about the specific needs of participants so that each person's problem can receive attention in later exercises. People, for example, with difficulties in noisy settings might receive specific attention during an exercise about socializing, while a person having problems with communication breakdowns might get more attention during exercises concerned with repair strategies. In addition, the leaders are also thinking about the level of ease with which participants identify and discuss issues. People's levels of openness are often indicative of the extent to which they are ready to deal with an issue and move on. It follows then that people who are more closed (rather than shy) about their experiences may need to be approached in a less direct fashion, giving them time to open up at first, rather than seeking to resolve issues. This would mean that for some individuals many of the exercises focus primarily on problem recognition and one would use them accordingly, while for others the issues would be about understanding and resolution. So while people are talking about their basic issues, the group leaders are thinking about key questions such as:

- What does the problem being presented by this person tell me about where they might be and what their issues and/or barriers might be?
- How emotionally difficult is it for them to speak about these issues?
- What indications are they giving out (speed of speech, flow of speech, folding of arms, sweat, blushing, anger, embarrassment, confidence, clarity, nervousness, etc.) about how they feel about such difficulties?
- What factors appear to predispose or reinforce the current behaviours?

- What strategies do people use presently?
- Watch out for self-reports of predisposing and reinforcing factors that justify inaction.

I trust that these points will become more apparent as we move through the materials. What is of primary importance at this stage is that the themes of mutual support and problem identification are continued throughout the rest of the programme as participants explore issues about the nature of hearing loss, its impact on their lives and options to manage the same. It will be apparent, however, that this exercise cannot be rushed and can readily take up to 45 minutes to 1 hour to complete. Participants have often been through a lot and this may be the first time they have had the opportunity to discuss such matters. This may be particularly so for partners who have had to provide an enormous amount of support to the Deafened person, over a very long period of time, often in traumatic circumstances. It is not uncommon, therefore, for some participants to express emotion at this time – some may cry. In such events, it is both important not to move on from such a person too quickly nor to linger too long. It is important to recognize and acknowledge the emotion, this expression of the level of difficulty of what the person is, or has been, going through and to provide support.

Crying is also an expression of emotional or tension release, and most people soon regain their composure. However, if people cannot regain their composure after a brief period, then the co-leader should see if they would like to leave the room for a while. If they would, the co-leader should go with them and provide support and assistance. For individuals requiring it, a referral may be made for psychotherapy as indicated. This may be especially important where the partner has supported the Deafened person through surviving suicidal ideation or other self destructive behaviours. It is important to remember here that while the crisis is usually long past, you are working with the emotional scars of a difficult time in someone's life.

The second objective of understanding the nature and consequences of a hearing problem is closely linked to the first. This objective is realized as participants and facilitators share their knowledge of hearing loss and some of its effects such as stress-related problems and reduced pleasure from social occasions. Information is not presented in a lecturing style. Rather, as new topics are introduced, the facilitator draws on the experience and knowledge of participants to explore and resolve issues, often constantly referring back to the materials participants identified in the first session. A series of social scenes, for example, are presented, where participants are asked to suggest the types of difficulties a hearing-impaired person might experience. Participants are then encouraged to identify particular difficulties and tensions that may be experienced within such a situation. Participants are then asked to identify strategies as to how such difficulties might best be managed or overcome. If a participant gets stuck, other participants are encouraged to suggest ideas that might be of assistance.

As shown in Figure 5.5, the group process begins to move from mere problem identification to problem identification and exploration. The exercise that works best in this setting is the *BBQ Party Exercise*. In this exercise, participants view a picture of a person's house, that of a friend or relative, and are told that they are to attend a party there. The picture of the party depicts a typical house layout but with an emphasis on the various communication hazards present such as noise, lighting, strange people and alcohol. During the exercise (which Deafened people and partners complete separately at first and then together) participants are asked to identify what they would do and how they would manage the problems that would confront them in such a situation. As with the first exercise, this second exercise is foundational and is therefore not to be rushed. The problem exploration phase has five goals of its own. These are to:

- identify current behaviours;
- explore current levels of awareness;
- explore the level of collaborative support present between client and partner;

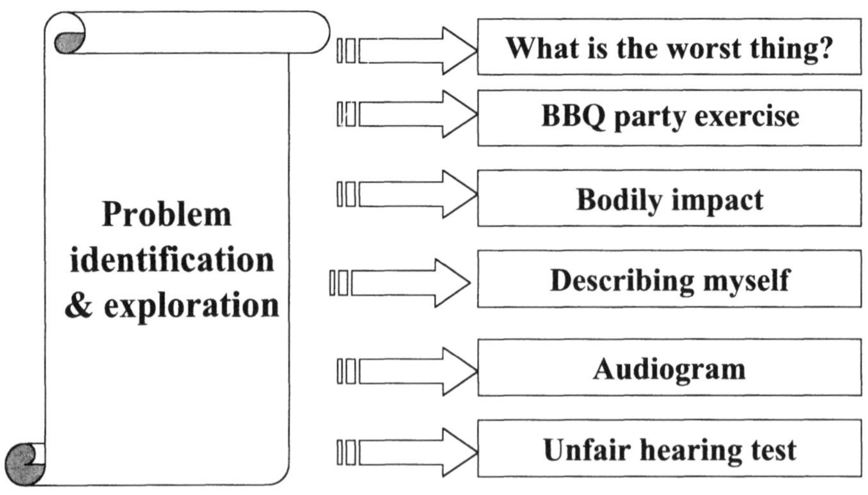

Figure 5.5: Overview of group programme 1.

- recognize the impact of such behaviours and awareness;
- examine to what extent hearing tactics are used, and their respective strengths and weaknesses.

The problem exploration stage seeks to draw from participants the contradictory reality of the traditional use of hearing tactics. The reality is like this: the clients, having been diagnosed with a hearing loss, a stigmatizing disability, are in turn told that every time they enter a conversation they are to:

- acknowledge their deafness;
- tell the communication partner where to sit/stand;
- adjust the lighting to suit their needs;
- modulate the speech of the communication partner;
- have things rephrased;
- seek clarification/confirmation and so on.

This is just not real. Deafened people often feel that they have no power or no legitimate reason to change the nature of interactions; that they are imposing their needs on to others. The purpose of this second phase of the workshop is, therefore, to draw out the fact that:

- difficulties occur;
- such difficulties reduce a person's quality of life;
- people often feel powerless to do much about these things;
- hearing tactics do not often work or that family and friends simply ignore one's needs;
- participants do not assert their needs and rights, feeling that it is wrong or selfish to do so;
- as individuals we tend to withdraw or isolate ourselves when confronted with such problems;
- such events are stressful;
- such difficulties are often unacknowledged.

The process of problem exploration then serves to legitimate the experience of living with hearing loss – 'it's not just me then', to enable participants to recognize the situations in which they have been embarrassed and to understand what it is about communication breakdown that is embarrassing. Specifically people think that they are seen as incompetent (i.e. stupid) as they cannot even manage the basic rituals of social interaction. So part of the problem exploration phase concerns itself with enabling participants to see that communication breakdown is not their fault, that it is not unique to them, that much of it has to do with taken-for-granted attitudes to deafness and disability.

So – what would people do when they go to a barbecue or similar party? Popular responses include:

- avoid going;
- leave early;
- withdraw, get frustrated or simply have a bad time;
- rely on the partner;
- get drunk;
- get embarrassed;
- corner someone and talk at them all night.

When partners return to the group they can confirm much of what has been said while actually being much better at identifying the nature of problems confronting their spouse. When such knowledge gaps emerge, it becomes apparent to what extent the Deafened clients lack insight into their own behaviours. In addition, partners may challenge those who have denied the things that they actually do. A Deafened person, for example, might say that he or she would of course go to the barbecue and have a good time. However, on hearing this, a partner may state that this is simply not true. This provides the group leader with the opportunity to draw out the issues of how difficult it is to deal with such situations and to reinforce the fact that this is why we are here as a group.

As part of problem exploration, it is important nonetheless, to have people focus on why it is that they may do nothing about the problems they confront. Reasons for inaction can include:

- not wanting to offend people;
- concern not to *rock the boat* or draw attention to oneself;
- continued reliance on the partner;
- easier to take the path of least resistance;
- fear and embarrassment.

Certainly a difficulty cited by many people is that outside of their own home they feel a lack of power to change things. Yet for many, it is actually with family and friends that they have a bad time socially. Oddly, in settings such as restaurants people are, to some extent, more inclined to stand up for themselves and their rights, but not at home. Yet as we will see later, it is often the way people manage these situations that is a core part of the problem. Overall, these factors reinforce the point that many Deafened people do not think it is right to ask people to change communication settings so that they can be included. It can be seen that the nature of everyday communication problems are neither easily recognized nor understood by Deafened people who often lack insight into their own behaviour, that socially they may readily become emotionally paralyzed and be either unable to negotiate change, lack a repertoire of problem resolution skills or not have the social ability to apply them in real settings. The key problem facing the Deafened person is this:

> The individual is not able to competently participate in everyday interactions without risking serious stigmatization and shame.

This is the problem that the group process seeks to address. Specifically, we seek to build up the client's communicative competence though skills-based training where such competencies are seen to consist of:

- knowledge – of what to do and how to do it;
- attitudes – it's OK to do it – it's good for me;
- communication skills – the capacity to put knowledge and attitudes into practice.

The enduring limitation in hearing rehabilitation to date is that there has been an over-emphasis on knowledge while failing to develop the clients' attitudes and interactive skills. It is one thing to practise making requests in the privacy of a clinic room in the presence of a sensitive and understanding therapist. It is an entirely different matter to assert oneself in front of strangers where one has to openly admit, perhaps for the first time, that one is deaf. Indeed, one of the most striking things that you will encounter in running these groups is the clients' inability to state, quickly, accurately and simply, their hearing loss and their needs in relation to it. Hence, the continued focus in the exercises on making 'I' statements (I am deaf, I need you to ...). What is most interesting though is the fact that the majority of people cannot simply make a coherent and accurate statement about their deafness – they are simply too embarrassed to do so.

So, having explored the issues of communication breakdown in some depth, the group is ready to move on to the third objective of the programme – *developing problem-resolving skills*. However, before doing so, it is important to give people a framework for doing so. This framework then forms the basis for all the teaching that will follow and the

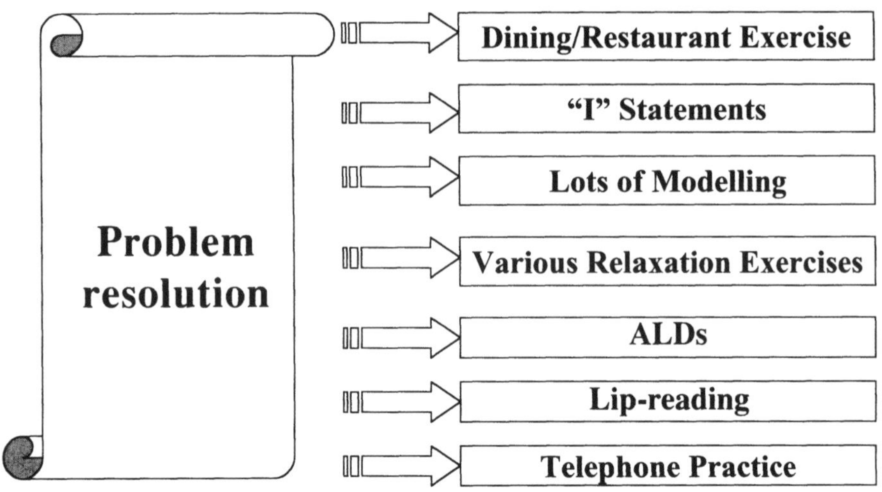

Figure 5.6: Overview of group programme 2. ALD = Assistive listening device.

training based on it results, in the emergence of a sense of pride and confidence in one's ability to manage in everyday settings and pivots on the development of a sense of who the person is (identity) and the values upon which such an identity is based.

I provide clients with a six-point guide to manage difficult social situations. These are:

- eliminate the problem before it arises (plan ahead);
- negotiate for an accessible communication environment;
- assert yourself (especially when things do not turn out as planned);
- reduce the problem (e.g. reduce background noise, set up quiet zone, improve lighting, etc.);
- put a barrier between the problem and yourself (i.e. move to another area; another room, etc.);
- put up with it or go home.

The important factor to work with here is to affirm that Deafened people need to set up rules for interaction that are going to work for them. This includes having a set of strategies for negotiating and developing confidence in their application. Certainly this paradigm is not a panacea for all communicative dilemmas that they will face. People will not always comply, be understanding or supportive or they may simply forget and often do. What it does do however is give the person a legitimate position of power from which to work, for if each of the 16–22 per cent of hearing-impaired people out there and their partners only engage one or two other people in accommodating them to these rules, before you know it half the population will be accommodating the needs of Deafened people.

To reinforce the learning process in phase three (which in fact now moves between problem exploration and resolution for the rest of the programme), participants have opportunities to practise effective communication strategies and the application of assertiveness skills within socially predictable settings. However, such problem-solving is not simply a matter of learning hearing tactics. It is about:

- developing knowledge and attitudes about the meaning of disability in the person's life;
- validating alternative communication practices;
- building self-concept;
- establishing a sense of personal pride based around a sense of communicative coherency and life continuity;
- learning to manage the cyclical interactive process of negotiation and emotional endeavour required to achieve satisfactory outcomes in problematic communication settings.

However, clients are not going to manage everyday communication problems with ease if they do not believe that it is acceptable to change the rules for communication. So an essential part of the group programme is reinforcing the fact that current behaviours, as demonstrated in the two introductory sessions, do not work well for clients, and then to establish new rules for communication.

In enabling clients to bring the ideas they learn about in the group programme into practice they need to use *'I' statements* – they are the key to effective outcomes. When asked to describe how they might respond to a difficult situation, clients will probably describe their behaviour of thinking in the third person (I would tell them to ...) and perhaps offer an anecdote to this effect. However, third person language serves as an emotionally protective barrier against the issue of acknowledging that one is deaf. Stories objectify the problem – it puts it out there, at a safe distance from people's lived experience.

Because deafness is stigmatizing it can be perceived by the individual, at a very deep level, to be personally threatening. Indeed, it has had dramatic consequences already in the people's lives. It is natural, therefore, to avoid drawing attention to it wherever possible and emotional energy may go into ensuring that people do not know of the deafness. Indeed, prior to the fuller onset of deafness, the clients may have actively avoided disclosing their deafness to anyone. How often do we hear even now, clients say proudly, that a person they were talking to did not even know that they were deaf. Yet, as was noted earlier, since a disclosure of deafness may have been perceived to be personally threatening, it may have also generated, particularly in the early days of deafness, an automatic response from the body's defence system, the sympathetic nervous system (increased heart rate, digestive shut down, muscle tension, adrenaline rush, etc).

Despite the demanding nature of this reactive process, the brain and the subconscious learnt that such a response, even if coupled with the shocked/numbed response of having to deal with such a personally threatening event, worked, where 'worked' meant that deafness was not disclosed or that one got through the troublesome interaction without being destroyed by the threat of their deafness. The brain is a dynamic and spontaneous organ. It works out that this set of responses (denial or minimization, effort, tactic and a psycho-physiological response), particularly when practised a number of times, enables the person to get by. In turn, the brain sets up an emotional-practical shortcut which is (technically) called a ***heuristic***. Then, every time the difficult situation, or anything vaguely similar to it, arises, the brain activates the shortcut. Where deafness is not readily acknowledged, less than ideal problem-solving comes into play and the person emotionally over-reacts in a manner not required by the situation at hand.

The use of 'I' statements serves not only to enable people to assert themselves, it also facilitates the dismantling of the heuristic that is at the heart of so many Deafened people's interactive difficulties. The use of the first person serves to facilitate the release of the emotional or psychic energy that has fuelled the formation of the heuristic in the first place. The sense of shame or embarrassment about being deaf begins to lift and a sense of pride begins to emerge. And because this release process can be achieved in part through a parallel process (one can experience an emotional shift simply by watching another person working through a similar issue – e.g. crying at the movies at a sad scene), problem-solving difficult situations in a group setting has the added benefit of providing repeated opportunities for the person to let go of the emotions that have become attached to their experience of deafness. 'I' statements then facilitate learning, behavioural change and emotional release. They help the development of new mental shortcuts for solving problems. It follows that, in addition to teaching the mind to let go, it is also important to teach the body to let go of its pent-up tensions that have resulted from repeated over-activations of the sympathetic nervous system. Hence the importance of teaching relaxation (discussed below).

Assertiveness

Many participants believe that they know how to assert themselves. While many are able to model being either passive, passive aggressive or just plain aggressive, most are not being assertive when they think they are and are in fact quite hostile to their communication partners. Within the programme there are a series of problematic social situations that require participants to practise being assertive, passive and aggressive. Work through these as they are outlined in the programme. As each person models a response to a situation, ask the other members of the group to give feedback to the person on their response. Was it assertive? Or was it passive and so on? Of course, acknowledge how difficult it is to assert oneself well, but also draw out over time that if in fact we have been aggressive, then perhaps this may in part be why communication breaks down.

The first problem resolution exercise is Harriet Kaplan and Scott Bailey's restaurant exercise. First, participants are led through the exercise in the usual manner, having respondents identify the communication hazards, the better tables to sit at and so on. The dynamics of the exercise are then reworked. Initially participants have identified where they would like to sit and why. The group leader then begins to role-play the situation, assuming that they are the *Maître de*. Placing participants at tables of their choosing, the Maître de/group leader in turn asks participants: would they be happy to sit at a prescribed table (usually one right in the worst spot for a Deafened person such as next to the piano)?:

- Would they sit there if directed to do so?
- How would they feel about having to sit there?
- What would happen to their body, their stress responses?
- What could they do to overcome these difficulties?

At this time participants will say things such as: I will sit there and put up with it; I would say nothing; and so on. It is important at this time to emphasize the point that they would be paying money to have a bad time, to be stressed or marginalized. Participants are asked if this is really what they want? Clearly it is not. Solutions to this situation are then role-played. By role-playing I do not mean getting up and walking about the room (though this is fine if people are comfortable to do so), but simply having people making requests, in keeping with their hearing loss is all that is required. This means enabling people to say, 'I am hearing-impaired/deaf and I will not be able to hear well at this table (or a similar statement is fine). I would like such and such a table.'

However, most people, when beginning 'I' statements will skirt around this issue, minimizing the extent of their deafness, by saying things such as – I'm a bit deaf. A bit deaf! This is poor communication and gives the communication partner the entirely wrong message. Clarify these issues with participants and work with them as they make correct and accurate statements about their hearing needs. Encourage other deafened participants to suggest solutions. Create dilemmas for individuals to solve. For example, a participant might appropriately request Table Six. Tell them that Table Six is taken – make them work for what they want – for if they will not make appropriate requests in the safety of the group – they certainly will not do so outside in the real world. Then, move on to identify strategic ways of avoiding problems using the hierarchy noted earlier (e.g. booking ahead, eating at restaurants that offer easy access to communication).

When you have finished the exercise, affirm and congratulate participants for their efforts, recognizing how difficult it may be for them, while reinforcing how many of these difficulties can be minimized or eliminated. Acknowledge that asserting oneself can be very difficult, noting that in the first instance communication partners may well assert themselves right back! This is fine. But clients often will say, 'Oh I tried that and it didn't work.' What they are often saying is that when the person asserted or aggressed back, they backed away or withdrew their request. Assertive behaviours often set up a series of interactions and negotiations, some of which are emotionally laden. Assertion therefore needs to be seen as a process that one goes through, a series of problem-solving dialogues and compromises that arise between two people until a common ground can be reached. A positive outcome cannot always be achieved. Assertiveness should not be seen as merely a one-off thing that either works or doesn't. For an excellent study of these issues see Robert Bolton's (1987) *People Skills – How to Assert Yourself, Listen to Others and Resolve Conflict*.

The problem resolution process commences slowly and works through a small number of exercises at some length. But then, as participants begin to get the idea of what is required, the remaining exercises are worked through with some speed as participants increase their competency. This work is in turn supplemented with information and personal support sessions. These include sessions concerned with the use of assistive listening devices. At the Link Centre, for example, these sessions are offered on a one-to-one basis, partly because their clients are quite severely hearing-impaired and a one-to-one model is found to be more effective. However, the Getty and Hetu model utilizes a group setting wherein participants can discuss their attitudes to and experiences with various devices.

Relaxation

Despite the fact that adjustment to hearing loss is stressful and physically demanding, few participants readily recognize the impact of disability on their physical and mental well-being. A core part of the rehabilitation process is concerned with enabling participants to recognize the effects of deafness on the body and the mind. Within the field of complementary therapies concerned with the body (e.g. acupuncture, massage, aromatherapy, chiropractic – especially the sacral-orbital technique – and homeopathy), it is well accepted that the signature of psychological trauma is stored with the cells of the body. Within western medicine the impact of unaddressed stress on physical and mental health is also well known. It is therefore critical to ensure that people with hearing loss and partners learn to recognize the manner in which stress manifests itself in their lives and then to develop strategies to address and reduce and/or eliminate it. It is insufficient simply to tell people that they need to relax – the psychosocial approach is concerned with enabling people to achieve this rehabilitation outcome. Obviously, while people who have developed more severe stress disorders may require ongoing help, the programme can serve to ensure that they identify and access interventions that are likely to be helpful to them.

Thus, during the group-process, individuals may be introduced to relaxation training, self-help books on stress management, the use of oil baths, aromatherapy massage, the use of essential oils, Tai Chi and the benefits of other complementary therapies. Most critically, while every aspect of personal care cannot be covered within a short programme, it is vital that participants leave the programme with knowledge and confidence in accessing at least some of these interventions. The Link Centre, for example, provides every participant with an aromatherapy massage, the University of Sydney programme (based on the Getty and Hetu model) offers relaxation training and information on alternative therapies while the Birmingham Centre for Deafened Adults offers a concurrent programme that teaches specific relaxation techniques.

More intensive psychotherapy may be of benefit to some participants as may relationship counselling. The Link Centre, the Birmingham Centre for Deafened Adults and the University of Sydney programmes offer participants one-to-one therapy with a qualified rehabilitation counsellor or psychologist.

Towards the end of the intervention, providers work with participants towards developing a personal action plan. Depending on the nature of the service, this plan may be a negotiation process between the provider and participants concerning ongoing work or counselling that may be done together. In services where the intervention is more 'one-off' in nature, the provider contracts with the service users to ensure that they will be able to achieve their rehabilitation outcomes once they move on, perhaps by providing referrals or relevant contacts. Figure 5.7 provides a summary of the change process.

Critique of the psychosocial approach

A group-based psychosocial approach to rehabilitation cannot be an exhaustive coverage of all issues pertaining to the rehabilitation of hearing impairment. Rather, the programme is based on principles of public health that are concerned with facilitating change in an individual's behaviour and attitudes concerning their hearing loss. As Getty and Hetu (1991) observe, it is about initiating a problem-solving process.

The psychosocial approach is, by its very nature non-expert, being centred on the clients' experiences for both problem definition and resolution. The problem-solving nature of the group process readily enables participants to reduce their dependence on professionals since they develop their own competencies in problem-solving. Given the ready use of professionally driven, expensive and highly technical interventions in the field of hearing impairment these days, an interactional approach to rehabilitation, that does not promote the uptake of any particular technology, is essential. It is only a start, a catalyst, an empowerment process that requires further effort and continuing work by the client – personal care is, a lifelong effort.

In summary then, the psychosocial approach draws together hearing-impaired people and their spouses, facilitates an empowerment process based on the attainment of information, support and skills development

- Getting the issue on the table – being stuck
- Identifying the personal/physical/social impact
- Defusing intensity through relaxation practice
- Building skills and confidence through problem-solving
- Psychological shift through identity building and role modelling

Figure 5.7: Overview of change process.

and initiates individual and social change based on an empowerment exchange process between the provider resourcing the process and the group, and within the group itself.

Evaluating outcomes

It is vital that psychosocial and technical aspects of any rehabilitation programme be evaluated. As per the objectives noted above, programme evaluation is concerned with measuring the extent to which the intervention improves participants' quality of life and reduces the experience of impairment and disability. To these ends, the evaluation protocol follows a pre/post design, using validated and reliable instruments wherever possible. Some of these instruments need to be generic measures of benefit. Generic measures are important as they enable providers to determine the overall extent to which interventions justify the use of public and insurer-provided monies.

Generic measures are the 'common language' or benchmarking tool of evaluation in health and disability services. However, such measures (e.g. the EuroQoL, Sintonen 15d) are often fairly insensitive to the subtle changes achieved in communication and relationship enhancement that result from hearing rehabilitation programmes. Thus a disability specific measure of outcomes is also required. Such measures may include the CPHI, the Code-Müller Protocols, the Glasgow Hearing Benefit Inventory and other hearing handicap scales. Ideally, the disability-specific measures would be validated against the better established generic measures of quality of life. Interestingly, the Assessment of Quality-of-Life measure (Hawthorne, Richardson and Osborne, 1999) has proved to be sensitive to outcomes in hearing rehabilitation programmes. Finally, socio-demographic items may also be collected. Where appropriate, these may include gender, age, marital status, employment status, occupation, current income and education. Where services are able to provide longer-term follow-up on client outcomes, these social indicators may provide a critical insight into the benefits of the programme provided. Included within this research effort, attention may also be given to measuring changes in self-concept and social confidence, issues often reported on by clients but seldom subjected to routine documentation.

CHAPTER 6

Engaging the client in a helping relationship

ANTHONY HOGAN AND CHRIS CODE

Preamble

This chapter continues the examination of the psychosocial support needs of people who receive cochlear implants. It shows that prospective clients and family members bring a range of expectations to the rehabilitation process. These expectations need to be identified and more adequately addressed within implant rehabilitation programmes. The chapter also demonstrates that in addition to being a clinical intervention, implant rehabilitation programmes have a socializing aspect, that of equipping Deafened adults to practise life as hearing people. Implantation places specific psychosocial demands on service users. These demands need to be acknowledged and managed systematically.

Introduction

We have already seen that disabilities such as deafness disrupt clients' lives. Things did not turn out the way they expected them to. Difficulties are experienced not just with hearing but with relationships, health, work and money. Deafened people approach rehabilitation clinics not just to regain their hearing, but to get their lives back into order. In this chapter we examine the experiences of Deafened people as they initially engage this implant process. On arrival at the implant clinic they set out, via implant technology, to be remade as hearing people. But this arrival is in fact a departure, the commencement of an odyssey, the journey of learning to live life as a Deafened person with a cochlear implant.

Expectations

Expectations surround the process of implantation. From the moment deafened individuals learn about the cochlear implant, they, as well as their family members, friends and clinicians, have expectations about how a particular person may fare with the device. In essence, this expectation builds upon the belief that implant technology *will* enable the reformation of the Deafened person. Unfortunately, such expectations do not always align and difficulties arise – difficulties that may be exacerbated by the practical experience of living with an implant. This shaping of expectations has in part been achieved through the extensive media coverage of cochlear implants promoted by manufacturers and clinics (Hogan, 1998b). In consequence, this has meant that implantation has come to be referred to as a miracle intervention. The miracle metaphor associated with cochlear implants poses immediate adjustment difficulties for the prospective implantee and the clinicians who will work closely with them.

Paula reflects on her thinking processes prior to implantation: 'I think, am I good enough to get a miracle?' A less than ideal outcome may mean that an implantee feels that they lack favour in the eyes of 'God', were not deserving of 'good luck' or that a negative outcome reflected poor karma. (An ideal outcome is one where the person communicates without the need for lip-reading.) The metaphor implicitly creates a barrier between the clinic and Deafened people because clients may come to feel unable to state what they really think about the implant – perceiving a less than ideal outcome as reflecting negatively on themselves or that they have let down the clinic. The metaphor also detracts from the physiological process being undertaken. An ossified cochlear or a damaged auditory nerve means that the amount of signal that can be delivered to the brain, even in ideal situations, is limited. By working within the physical confines of the process at hand, and by avoiding unhelpful metaphors, clinics immediately become more able to manage the various expectations that clients may bring to this process.

Most clinicians would agree that extensive client and family education prior to implantation is essential to a good outcome. However, as Rick's experience shows, the provision of information in itself may be not be rationally taken in by the prospective candidate. Despite having been made aware of the limitations of cochlear implants, Rick entered the programme with an enduring hope:

> ... they explain it to ya that you're never gonna be like normal hearing and everything like that. (*But you hoped anyway?*) Well, it's always there [laughing] isn't it! Like you might sit down and hoping to win the lotto, like that hope! Like ya say, if you've got a battler with no money around or anything. Well he's sitting around, well he's hoping. He's filling out his coupon, and he's hoping this is the day. That's how I think it is when you're deaf. Like this. You're hoping, next week, next week.

Implicit in clients' motivation to have a cochlear implant, are personal and social expectations about what they will be able to do when *they can hear again*, and what sort of people they will become. Rick, for example, wanted to have an implant to make up to his wife for being deaf; in losing his hearing, he felt he had let her down. He also wanted to be able to know when people were at the front door; a problem readily solved by a flashing door light. A cochlear implant was not going to solve Rick's feelings of guilt associated with his disability. Jack and Liz, on the other hand, had different motivations. Jack needed communication for work and personal interests (such as listening to music), while Liz was very isolated and needed basic communication to facilitate daily living.

What one hopes to be as a result of implantation then serves to influence people's motivation and perceptions of themselves throughout the rehabilitation process. It is important, during the pre-implant work-up, to work with clients to help them describe the sorts of goals they might have for their communication. This ideal is fraught with difficulties as potential implantees may be inclined to tell the clinician what they *think* they should say in order to pass successfully through the assessment process. Identifying client expectations then becomes part detective work, as one sifts through the clients' life experiences prior to and post deafness, in order to identify the things they have lost and seek to have restored. We need to identify who they were prior to deafness, the sorts of things they liked to do, and then identify the range of skills and abilities they'd like to get back again. So, the question *'why would you like an implant?'* becomes redundant as it only produces a predictable answer – 'because I'm deaf.'

Clinicians are experienced in taking factual case histories from their clients. In preparing a candidate for a possible implant, the clinician seeks to develop a *theorized case history* of the client. In taking this history the clinician seeks to identify and summarize key events that occurred within the client's life as related to the motivation to have an implant and, based on this information, develop a plan to manage the client's psychosocial needs, and information counselling requirements for the rehabilitation process. When taking this type of history, probably at the initial interview, the first question to be put then is an open-ended one:

WOULD YOU MIND TAKING A FEW MOMENTS TO TELL ME ABOUT WHAT HAPPENED TO YOUR HEARING?

Every Deafened person has a story to tell. The types of stories that result from this question can be found in Chapter 2. They are quite long and contain a lot of very useful information, so adequate time needs to be set aside to take the history properly. At this time, clients' experiences of other rehabilitation processes can also be noted. This information is important as it gives an indication of their experiences with previous health professionals, any concerns they might have about being *let down* or frustrated within the helping process and expectations they might have about how you will work with them:

> COULD YOU PLEASE TELL ME ABOUT OTHER SERVICES THAT YOU USED TO HELP WITH YOUR HEARING. WHAT WERE THEY AND HOW DID YOU FIND THEM?

Taking a history such as this can take up to an hour, so allow for this amount of time. It is expected that during this interview clients may express emotion as they recall the traumatic events that have brought them to your rooms. This is fine. Crying is part of the healing process and it is important to allow people this grieving time. It is not always necessary to say anything, but a comforting and accepting presence is useful to clients as it signals to them that you recognize the validity of what they have experienced. Most people will not cry for long, although I once had a client who cried for two hours following the loss of residual hearing. Crying is often a process of emotional release. However, if crying persists over several interviews, a referral for psychotherapy may be indicated.

At this stage in the engagement interview you will have some knowledge about:

- what clients have lost;
- what they possibly desire from your clinic;
- their experiences with rehabilitation providers;
- their ability to manage frustrations;
- their capacity to work on themselves in a consistent fashion.

Following the development of this understanding, move on to asking the client and partner what they expect from the rehabilitation process, particularly from implantation. However, an indirect approach is again indicated here so as not to script the client into telling you the obvious and to avoid enabling the client to tell you what they think you want to hear. The client is not the only person with expectations to be managed. Partners also have expectations and it is important to engage both of them in the process so that the best outcome can be achieved.

In order to avoid clients locking themselves into circular arguments and with a view to accurately identifying the needs of clients and partners, a client-centred counselling protocol is indicated. The Code-Müller Protocols (CMP) are a method for working with clients, in a collaborative fashion, so that their psychosocial rehabilitation needs can be addressed adequately.

The Code-Müller Protocols (CMP)

The CMP were originally developed to complement a client-centred approach to the rehabilitation of adults with acquired communication disorders such as aphasia. This approach emphasizes the important role played by the client *and* significant others (SOs) in their lives and in their rehabilitation process. The approach pivots on the assumption that outcomes from rehabilitation programmes might be enhanced by focusing on the hopes, expectations and perceptions that clients, their partners and the professionals held for the rehabilitation process. The CMP does this through the use of a simple questionnaire of ten items designed to gain information on the individual perceptions of psychosocial adjustment by the client, and those personally and/or professionally involved with them.

A range of studies have shown that the CMP can provide useful information for counselling with aphasic, dysarthric, right-hemisphere damaged and laryngectomy clients and their relatives (Code, Khanbha and Mattiazzo, 1996; Hemsley and Code, 1996; Herrmann and Wallesch, 1989). The primary objective of the CMP is to create a forum wherein the individual client and others (SOs and any number of health professionals working with the client) can compare perceptions concerning the clients' progress in adjusting to their acquired disability. This forum can yield valuable information about competing and contrasting goals, priorities and client/practitioner barriers within the rehabilitation process, that cannot be obtained from other physiological or medical sources.

The ten items which make up the version revised for use with people with acquired hearing loss, require the person completing it to rate the clients, on a five-point scale, on their: ***ability to do work, communicate, be independent, socialize, cope with disability related depression, frustration and embarrassment, pursue hobbies, speak to strangers and make new friends***. This list reflects a small yet salient range of psychosocial factors related to abilities to form close relationships, overcome feelings of self-pity, and to adjust to communication difficulties (for a full list of items as adapted for those people with profound hearing loss, see Figure 6.4).

This short protocol is not meant to provide a comprehensive profile of the individual's psychosocial state. The questions are considered to represent no more than a sampling of psychosocial opportunities and scenarios. With the 5-point scale the neutral position (stay the same) always scores 3, 'get much worse' scores a 1 and 'improve a lot' scores a 5, as follows:

1 = get much worse	2 = get a little worse	3 = stay the same
4 = improve a little	5 = improve a lot	

The questionnaire is given to the client, and any significant others (SOs) in the client's life – such as spouse, relatives, carers, as well as any professionals involved with the client, especially any key people working with the client. Everyone is asked to complete the questionnaire using the five-point scale to rate change on the ten items. The main product of the CMP is a measure of optimism or confidence about the future which can be simply obtained by adding scores together for an individual (e.g. higher scores indicate higher optimism). However, optimism measured by the CMP appears to interact with chronicity (time since onset of impairment) and emotional and psychosocial states (Herrmann and Wallesch, 1990; Code and Muller, 1992). Responses to various questions (completed by any respondent) can be examined individually or collectively as a basis for counselling. Respondents for example, may all agree that the client's *ability to cope with frustration due to hearing problems* appears to be getting worse (i.e. their *ability to cope with frustration* was rated as decreasing a little or a lot). The CMP offers a useful base for pre-implant counselling as the clinician can ask the client or SO specific questions concerning their expectations, that can in turn be used to counsel the client about what the implant can and cannot do for their hearing and to prepare them for learning new communication skills and assertiveness strategies. For example:

> I SEE THAT YOU THINK THAT YOUR ABILITY TO COPE WITH FRUSTRATIONS DUE TO HEARING PROBLEMS WILL GREATLY IMPROVE IN THE FUTURE. CAN YOU TELL ME ABOUT SOME OF THE FRUSTRATIONS YOU ARE CURRENTLY EXPERIENCING?

When listening to the client's response, the clinician is seeking to assess the nature of problems experienced by the client in order to identify those difficulties which the implant cannot resolve. It is important then, not to say much at this stage of the interview, but to continue asking probing questions, as the client may realize that there are a variety of issues that the implant will not resolve and therefore become defensive and close up. Other questions would follow on in a similar fashion:

> I SEE TOO THAT YOU THINK THAT YOUR ABILITY TO COPE WITH EMBARRASSMENT DUE TO HEARING PROBLEMS WILL ALSO GREATLY

IMPROVE IN THE FUTURE. CAN YOU TELL ME ABOUT A TIME RECENTLY WHEN YOU FELT EMBARRASSED ABOUT YOUR (PARTNER'S) HEARING?

I SEE THAT YOU THINK THAT YOUR ABILITY TO MAKE NEW FRIENDS WILL GREATLY IMPROVE IN THE FUTURE. CAN YOU TELL ME ABOUT SOME OF THE FRUSTRATIONS YOU ARE CURRENTLY EXPERIENCING?

WHAT HOBBIES ARE YOU INTERESTED IN? HOW DOES YOUR HEARING PROBLEM PREVENT YOU FROM PURSUING THESE INTERESTS?

Once you have completed this process of information gathering, you may make summary statements about the clients' needs and assure them that they will be addressed within the rehabilitation process. As well, it is timely to emphasize that specific problems (note them) will not be resolved, or fully resolved by the implant and that communication therapy will also be required.

Congruence

Congruence refers to the extent of agreement between parties about future predictions on the client's psychosocial adjustment. It is a reflection of the agreement experienced by all parties and can be examined, compared and contrasted on the CMP. Incongruence may arise because the client or partner becomes impatient with the rehabilitation process, or because the client fails to realize that some problems are social, rather than technical in nature. A *Perceptual Congruence Quotient* (PCQ) can be readily calculated by comparing the sets of scores that individuals produce (see Code and Müller, 1992). The PCQ is a reflection of overall congruence between all parties. Most commonly these will be the basic triad: the clinician with the client; the clinician with the SO; the client with the SO.

The clinician can construct profiles where both optimism and congruity can be graphically expressed and more easily understood by all concerned and further analysis can be done to widen the value of the information gained from the questionnaire. Most notably, partners tend to have very high expectations and clinicians tend to have lower expectations for the implant process, so it is important to counsel the partners about their expectations so that they are more able to support the clients through the post-implant adjustment process.

Setting priorities in rehabilitation

In addition to differences arising between various clinicians, clients and others over perceptions of progress in rehabilitation, differences may also arise over the relative importance of CMP-R items and therefore, the planning of rehabilitation programmes. The Multiple Attribute Utility Technique (Herrmann and Wallesch, 1990; Code and Muller, 1992) can be applied with the CMP-R. The Multiple Attribute Utility Technique (MAUT) enables clinicians and others to sort out priorities in the rehabilitation process through a process of ranking and weighting CMP-R items.

Ranking and weighting have specific clinical functions. Ranking allows for the ordering of items with regard to the importance each item may have for the clinician, client or SO. For example, a clinician may conclude that enabling a client to *cope with frustration due to hearing problems* is more important than developing *skills for speaking to strangers*. Weighting, on the other hand, identifies the extent to which a clinician or client thinks one issue is more important than another – weighting the items highlights the relative relevance of an item compared with other items. For example, the clinician may think that developing skills for speaking to strangers is the least important issue within the rehabilitation programme and that *hobby skills* is more important but not nearly as important as *enabling the client to get to work*. Once items have been ranked and weighted by clinicians, clients and SOs, perceptions on relevance as well as item congruence can be utilized in counselling and planning within a client-centred rehabilitation process.

Scoring the MAUT

The MAUT is a strategy that can be used in conjunction with your clients to set priorities for rehabilitation. There are at least two ways to set these priorities. We will commence with the longer and more methodological procedure first. If you are not interested in this then skip to the next page where a

- 1 Cope with frustration
- 2 Embarrassment
- 3 Independence
- 4 Socialization
- 5 Hobbies
- 6 Speak to strangers
- 7 Work
- 8 Depression
- 9 Make new friends
- 10 Ability to communicate

Figure 6.1: Ranked CMP items – one clinician's rankings.

simpler method for priority setting can be found. In order to set preferences for what will be done in therapy and for how long, CMP items are initially ranked in order of importance from 1 to 10, 1 being most important (Figure 6.1). The respondents then weight each item in multiples of ten, starting with the least important item which is weighted ten. The respondents then weight the item ranked 9 in multiples of ten, depending on their perceptions of its relevance. So the item rated 9 (in this example see Figure 6.2) may be weighted 50, compared with the item ranked 10. The respondent may, however, weight the 9th item ranked, 300 or 3,000.

In the worked example in Figures 6.1 and 6.2, the clinician working with the deafened adult completed the procedure. In Figure 6.1, it can be seen that the clinician ranked *make new friends* and then *ability to communicate* as the least important items. In Figure 6.2, she weighted these items 50 and 10, respectively. However, she then weighted the next least important item (*depression*) 4 times higher than the previous item (200 verses 50). At the other end of the scale she weighted item 8 (*cope with frustration* – ranked number one) as the most relevant with a weighting of 2000. Once again, there is no upper limit in the weighting process. Finally, a percentage weighting for each item is calculated by dividing the score for each item by the total of weights. In Figure 6.3, weightings have been calculated on the average of the clinician's scores. The weighting of items on the CMP have been compared in a range of professional groups, including speech language pathologists, physiotherapists, occupational therapists, neuropsychologists and neurologists. Differences in weightings on CMP items between professionals have been found (Herrmann and Wallesch, 1990; Hemsley and Code, 1996, Herrman and Code, 1996).

As an alternative to the MAUT procedure, some clinicians have found it simpler to use the idea of having 100 units to spend on therapy and then

•	1	Cope with frustration	•	1	2000
•	2	Embarrassment	•	2	1800
•	3	Independence	•	3	750
•	4	Socialization	•	4	700
•	5	Hobbies	•	5	600
•	6	Speak to strangers	•	6	450
•	7	Work	•	7	400
•	8	Depression	•	8	200
•	9	Make new friends	•	9	50
•	10	Ability to communicate	•	10	10

Figure 6.2: Weighted CMP items.

• 1	Cope with frustration	• 1	2000–29%
• 2	Embarrassment	• 2	1800–26%
• 3	Independence	• 3	750–11%
• 4	Socialization	• 4	700–10%
• 5	Hobbies	• 5	600–9%
• 6	Speak to strangers	• 6	450–6%
• 7	Work	• 7	400–5%
• 8	Depression	• 8	200–3%
• 9	Make new friends	• 9	50–1%
• 10	Ability to communicate	• 10	10–0%
			6930–100%

Figure 6.3: Weighted CMP items.

to allocate these units, in order of importance (weight) across the 10 items. Either way, one ends up with a percentage of time available allocated to each issue of concern to the client and/or therapist.

The CMP were revised for use with adults within hearing rehabilitation programmes (CMP-R), particularly cochlear implant clinics. The revisions entailed relatively simple adjustment of the wording of items to be appropriate to the needs of deafened adults.

Hook-up, switch-on and the management of dampened expectations

Following implantation and wound healing, implantees and family members look forward with excitement to the day when the implant is switched on. The time when a speech processor is turned on has a variety of names around the world. These include hook-up, switch-on, start-up and initial programming. In addition to the technical process, two other processes need to be managed at 'switch on'. First is the social process (what the family expects the client to be able to do versus what the person will actually be able to do); second is the personal process (the client's reaction to switch-on and their sense of self-esteem as they prepare to confront an expectant world). Dominic's partner vividly describes their experience of switch-on day. (It should be noted here that pseudonyms for partners and other family members have not been used in order to relieve the reader's burden of trying to remember too many names or too much irrelevant detail. It is not to extinguish such people from the text or to deny the important contribution such people make in the lives of deafened adults.) Her description stands in stark contrast to the process portrayed in the media where the family gathers round to share in this intensely personal moment:

> I mean it was a pretty stressful thing. It was a big decision and you've got that waiting period then, before they go and switch you on. And you don't know what it's going to be like. I mean it's – imagine how scary it must have be for the person who's gone through all of this, and they're gunna go down and get switched on. Well, you don't send somebody off by themselves to ... do that! You know you want to be there – you want to support them but also – I mean my idea was that well if he's gunna hear something, God – he's gunna hear us first!

Service users have an expectation about the switch-on experience that is influenced by media portrayals of cochlear implantation – this is the miracle moment that they have been waiting for. Invariably televised portrayals depict a smiling yet stunned implantee expressing a bemused look as the first sound is pulsed through the device by the audiologist. A smiling surgeon and family look on. (Clinics have to accept some responsibility for the media portrayal of the implant. Afterall, TV news teams do not loiter in the halls of implant clinics hoping that the newest, youngest, or oldest ever implantee is about to be switched on. These media events are co-organized by clinics – they therefore have a role in determining what is published. For a more complete analysis of the media's portrayal of cochlear implants see Hogan (1998a).) For prospective candidates, this is what implantation is supposed to be all about – it was what Dominic's family were waiting for. Of course, Dominic's family's experience of switch-on was quite different. Dominic's wife continues:

> So OK, I arrange for the children to have the day off school because we like to do these things as a family and I think that it was very important for them too. So you know, they'd take the day off school and I'd take the day off work and we'd all go down to ... see the audiologist, who keeps us sitting around waiting for hours. Well not hours – but a while. We all go in you know. And she virtually told us to 'piss off!' you know. Like what are you doing here?!

Conversely, when Jack was implanted, his clinic was really excited about the event. Yet for him, the clinic's excitement about the technology completely exceeded his experience of the switch-on process, which was in his terms, a disappointment:

> So umm, all the electrodes work. They say 'fine!' see. So they put the programme processor and turn it on and expecting me to be delighted; and this

> is (not) different from other people – I've compared! What I heard was nothing like normal sound at all, it was just like birds twittering. It was all high pitched nonsense. I was dismayed. I thought how can I make any sense of that?

Implantees describe the first sounds heard with the implant as robotic, tinny and unnatural. Implantees are advised that this is normal and that they have to learn to hear with the implant. Such learning results from hard work and time. Although some people may immediately understand speech when the processor is switched on, the majority do not. With earlier speech processors, one had to work for several months simply to get used to the noises emitted by the implant; for people with newer processors, useable benefit appears within one to two months. Nonetheless, Fiona's description of the process shows just how hard learning to use an implant can be:

> There was another young lass. She was done not long after me and the next time I saw her I said how are you going with this. 'Terrible!' She said 'It's terrible'. She said 'I won't wear it ... She put it away and I said look 'You've got to persevere.' I said 'put it on when you get up in the morning and take it off at night'. Next time I saw her I said how are you going. She never takes it off. It took her six months to learn to keep it on.

Following switch-on, the brain has to learn to decipher the noise as sound. Training begins with learning how to differentiate between words of the same length and equal syllables (e.g. hot dog, football). Respondents report having to spend many hours learning to communicate and that it may be quite some time after implantation before one might converse with some ease. Liz, for example, received one of the earliest devices available, and it took 18 months before the implant offered her communication rather than noise.

Reconciling reality

For Rick implantation resulted in disappointment. He thought the device sounded like chipmunks and he felt that it never offered him the level of communication he had once enjoyed:

> I find the only thing I've got against it, is the clarity. The clarity like as far as anything else is concerned, like I can hear a plane, took me a long time to figure it out what the noise was, but I can hear a plane going over the home. Ah, but that sort of thing I could never hear before. I sit there, I couldn't hear the telephone ring. If I got this on [speech processor] I hear the telephone ring. I know the telephone's ringing. Like doors slamming. It takes a long time to pick up what it is to sort of balance what's going on. That takes a long time. But, I

> don't think like in meself that I've got any real complaints about it. Um ... I mean to say it's just a disappointment. Not a complaint. You know what – it's a disappointment, I wouldn't complain about it. Like [they] just asked me once did I just want to leave it [the speech processor] there – you know and forget about it. But I thought oh well, I keep it going. (Rick)

The implant provided Rick with an environmental input and made lip-reading easier – a good outcome for a person who had had no hearing for many years. But he was disappointed with the result. It was nothing like the sensation of sound as he remembered it, nor did it resolve his domestic problems. Issues with his wife still needed to be resolved and he still needed a flashing door light. Rick's disappointment was predictable. Effective psychological counselling prior to implantation may have addressed Rick's feelings of guilt and resolved marital tensions, therein preparing Rick with more realistic expectations as to what might be achieved with a cochlear implant. Such counselling could have also been informed by data based on the experiences of other people within the implant programme.

Learning to use the implant is a slow process. Paula has been implanted for six years, is on her second speech processor and relies on lip-reading and the sound of her implant for receptive communication. Her newer processor provided her with clearer and therefore easier communication, but it is still not a perfect process:

> I can sort of hear it. If you told me you were going to say something, I close my eyes. I can write down how much I got. I won't get it 100% right. But I'm not complaining!

Learning to hear presents as a difficult and fickle process:

> I remember the first time [I heard] after the bionic ear, I closed my eyes a lot – to listen. And the priest said the Our Father and I said Lord I can hear! And then he turned around and said something else and I didn't know a word he was saying (Paula).

Therapy can take a long time and outcomes at times appear intangible. At one time Paula completed a 'hearing' test and apparently responded correctly, even though she had little idea of the fact. For implantees, the process is demanding, confusing and stressful. Following the completion of such sessions, Paula remarked that she often had to go away somewhere and cry; she simply could not pick up what was being said to her. Progress with the implant is idealized in the ability to listen and understand words without lip-reading; for example by being able to use the telephone. This in itself becomes a source of stress for implantees because one has spent so long developing communication skills like lip-reading. It is traumatic to realize that a hard-earned and valued skill will now readily be lost in the name of progress.

Following implantation, the clinicians find themselves in a new process of mentally calibrating the client with the device, getting them used to each other and working towards facilitating the development of speech and hearing while gradually bringing the client to the realization that the outcome is the outcome. Certainly disappointment can be minimized by properly counselling the client prior to implantation and by providing a well structured and intensive programme of auditory training immediately following switch-on.

Expect practical limitations

The implant does not eliminate everyday communication problems associated with being deaf. Table 6.1 provides an overview of the extent of communication and relational difficulties experienced by implantees. Those who have retained family and broader relationships rate them positively. Less positive is the fact that implantees feel less valued by family and friends because of their deafness (80% and 73%). Everyday communication strategies used by deafened adults (such as rephrasing statements, asking people to repeat statements), elicit annoyance from family and friends, leaving the implantee feeling frustrated. These broader difficulties indicate once again the need for family or group-based rehabilitation interventions (discussed in the following chapters).

Table 6.1: Social and communication difficulties experienced by implantees (n = 129)

Issue	*Responded often/always (%)*
Feel less confident because of hearing loss	57
Feel left out in groups	36
Feel frustrated when needing to ask family to repeat	65
Friends annoyed when asked to repeat	76
TV at preferred volume annoys family	22
People I live with do not understand what hearing loss means	26
My friends would like me more if I could hear	73
Family annoyed when asked to repeat	76
I do not get on well with everyone in family	18
My family would love me more if I could hear	80
I am not happy at work/school	19
Feel frustrated when needing to ask friends to repeat	30
I don't get on well with friends	20

Source: Questions adapted from Getty and Hetu (1991) and Weinberg and Sterrit (1991).

In addition to encountering day-to-day communication problems, implantees point out that they frequently encounter problems using the technology. When the processor fails, it needs to be returned to the factory for repairs. Breakdowns are not uncommon and most clinics carry at least one processor for 'loan out' while a client's processor is being repaired. The 'loan out' scheme works well provided that only one implant is broken at a time. Attachment cords, belt clips and microphones break or can be lost. The external microphone is held in place on the user's head by a magnet. The magnet has a tendency to 'jump' onto metal objects such as the door of the refrigerator! Power supply to the speech processor is an ongoing problem. When the battery goes dead, the speech processor simply stops operating. In older processors (and there are still many in use) the batteries can go flat without warning. Newer processors can demand high levels of power, creating an on-going cost to the user, even when rechargeable units are utilized. Technical repairs are also expensive, costing implantees an estimated $400 per year (Carter and Hailey, 1995). Some clients have reported that the implant can pick up interference from magnetic fields such as those produced by power lines while others have noted that the device can set off security alarms in department stores. When outside, the microphone is sensitive to the wind, resulting in further distortions of sound and discomfort. The technology is sensitive to water and cannot be used with water sports or aerobics (due to sweat). Some speech processors can be worn around the waist and can fall off – not an unusual or infrequent event in the lavatory.

Implant technology has undergone significant changes since such devices became commercially available more than ten years ago (Hollows et al., 1995). In consequence, implantees will find themselves living with a redundant speech processor within three years of implantation. Given the demonstrated advances in the technology, it is evident that implantees would want newer processors as they become available. Prospective candidates need to know that additional costs are likely to be incurred. Alternatively, clinics need to identify additional resources in order to enable implantees to acquire improved processors as they become available.

Mapping expectations

It is evident from this discussion that service user expectations play a critical role in the success of any implant rehabilitation process. Such expectations need to be managed from the moment patients arrive at the clinic for even the most basic of consultations. The management of rehabilitative expectations requires an engagement with client and family where specific psychological as well as information needs are addressed. As part of a pre-implant programme, prospective service users (especially those who have been deaf for a long time) need to be involved in the development of their own rehabilitation plan. The purpose of such a plan is to ensure that strategies are put in place to address the various psychosocial aspects of the rehabilitative process identified here (e.g. Table 6.1).

The programme would ensure that the prospective service users understand what it is they are likely to gain from implantation (e.g. assistance with environmental noises; aided verbal communication). They would be informed about any physiological problems that may result in a poor outcome (e.g. ossified cochlear; long duration of deafness, poor existing lip-reading skills) and they would participate in discussions concerning identity and the impact of having a disability. This would in part include talking to other implantees as well as deafened adults who chose not to proceed to implantation. In addition to auditory training, the plan would also encompass post-implant education, social skills training and structured sessions of peer interaction, in order to enable implantees to situate their experiences alongside that of other implantees and to make sense of the overall process in which they have been involved. The mere provision of written information is insufficient – as Rick demonstrated, it is easy for clients to idealize any prospective outcome. Facilitated discussion groups, audiological counselling protocols (such as the Code-Müller Protocol – Revised), and psychological counselling all form part of an integrated implant rehabilitation programme, as do strategies for evaluating progress and for managing inevitable tensions that may arise between service users and clinics.

Concluding remarks

People using cochlear implant rehabilitation programmes approach implantation with high expectations and differing needs. These needs and expectations can be readily identified and addressed within the rehabilitation process. Original models for implant-based hearing rehabilitation programmes provided for the management of psychosocial aspects of the rehabilitation process (Clark et al., 1987). In the transition from research to clinically-based programmes, this aspect of rehabilitation has been largely omitted. Client and family perspectives on implant rehabilitation presented here demonstrate the complexity of psychosocial processes associated with cochlear implantation. It is time to recognize these needs and to structure future interventions to include psychosocial issues so that the best possible outcomes can be achieved.

CODE-MÜLLER PROTOCOLS				
Tick the most appropriate answer. Please answer all questions.			Date:	
Client's Name:			Clinician's Name:	
Name of Person Completing Questionnaire:			Total CMP Score:	
1. Do you think the ability to work (or do school work) will:-				
get much worse	get a little worse	stay the same	Improve a little	Improve a lot
2. Do you think that with more therapy the ability to communicate will:-				
get much worse	get a little worse	stay the same	improve a little	improve a lot
3. Do you think dependence on others will:-				
get much worse	get a little worse	stay the same	improve a little	improve a lot
4. Do you think the ability to meet friends socially will:-				
get much worse	get a little worse	stay the same	improve a little	improve a lot
5. Do you think the ability to cope with depression due to the hearing problem will:-				
get much worse	get a little worse	stay the same	improve a little	improve a lot
6. Do you think the ability to follow interests and hobbies will:-				
get much worse	get a little worse	stay the same	improve a little	improve a lot
7. Do you think the ability to speak to strangers will:-				
get much worse	get a little worse	stay the same	improve a little	improve a lot
8. Do you think the ability to cope with frustration due to the hearing problems will:-				
get much worse	get a little worse	stay the same	improve a little	improve a lot
9. Do you think the ability to make new personal friendships will:-				
get much worse	get a little worse	stay the same	improve a little	improve a lot
10. Do you think the ability to cope with embarrassment due to the hearing problem will:-				
get much worse	get a little worse	stay the same	improve a little	improve a lot

Figure 6.4: Code-Müller Protocols.

Code-Muller Protocols – Revised
MAUT (Multiple Attribute Utility Technique) Analysis

Instructions: Rank the items listed below in order of importance from your own point of view. Give a rank of 1 for the most important through to 10 for the least important. You should then weight the items as follows: give 10 to the least important item (i.e. the item you ranked 10th) and then assign values to the other items according to their relative importance in multiples of 10. For example, you may decide that the item you ranked 9th is 4 times more important for you than the item you ranked 10th, so you give it a weighting of 40. You decide that the item you ranked 8th is only just more important than the items you ranked 9th, so you give it a weighting of 50.

Name/Initials of person completing MAUT: Date:	Rank	Weight	Percentage Weighting
1. Do you think that your ability to work (or do school work) will:-			
2. Do you think that with more therapy your ability to communicate will:-			
3. Do you think that your dependence on others will:-			
4. Do you think that your ability to enjoy meeting friends socially will:-			
5. Do you think your ability to cope with depression due to hearing problems will:-			
6. Do you think your ability to follow current interests and hobbies will:-			
7. Do you think your ability to speak to strangers will:-			
8. Do you think your ability to cope with frustration due to hearing problems will:-			
9. Do you think your ability to make new personal friendships will:-			
10. Do you think your ability to cope with embarrassment due to hearing problems will:-			
Totals			

Figure 6.5: Code-Müller Protocols – revised.

CMP – PCQ

	1	2	3	4	5
Q1					
Q2					
Q3					
Q4					
Q5					
Q6					
Q7					
Q8					
Q9					
Q10					

○ Client
□ Partner
* Clinician

Figure 6.6: CMP: Perceptual Congruence Quotient.

Chapter 7

Structuring interventions

Preamble

Deafened adults present at audiological clinics for 'help' with their hearing difficulties. It is now evident that some of these difficulties have their basis in social and interpersonal difficulties, the resolution of which cannot be found within a technological fix but through interpersonal counselling, assertiveness training, communication skills development, and through the effective use of assistive devices. A certain motivation brings the client (and partner) to present at a clinic. It is essential to work with clients to explore the nature of this motivation so that their deeply felt needs can be matched with an appropriate intervention. Where high technology is involved, clients will present in the expectation that this technology will 'fix up' their problems and that this outcome will be achieved in a timely fashion. Part of the challenge of engaging with the client is to approach motivation and expectation indirectly, for any direct discussion about motivation locks the clinician into the client's rationality. An example of directness illustrates the point:

Clinician: Why are you interested in a cochlear implant?
Client: Because I am profoundly deaf – I can't hear; the implant will help me to hear again.
Clinician: Of course you realize that the implant will not give you back perfect hearing – in fact it may be an aid to hearing – you will probably still need to lip-read.
Client: Yes I know this – but any improvement would be very helpful to me.

It is an obvious and circular argument – a person is deaf – implants 'fix' deafness – I want an implant. Yet as we have seen from the previous chapters, the waters of motivation are often muddied with other more complex issues than an individually oriented, technology-based model of rehabilitation can address solely – there's a world out there that has to be reckoned with – with or without the use of technology.

In order to avoid locking into a circular argument with clients and with a view to identifying their rehabilitation needs accurately, a client-centred counselling protocol, as identified in Chapter 6, is indicated. In this chapter, strategies for engaging the client into a problem-solving approach are discussed and developed. To achieve this, the process of rehabilitation needs to be structured into phases that:

- reflect the issues confronting stakeholders within the process;
- facilitate the management of clients as they *move through* their rehabilitation programme.

Structuring the rehabilitation process is then about developing *signposts* that indicate to clients:

- where they are up to within the rehabilitation process;
- the stages that lie ahead;
- that the process has a clear beginning, a middle and an end.

Such structuring does not prescribe the rehabilitation process, rather it frames it. The experienced clinician readily knows that rehabilitation can often be three steps forward and two steps backwards.

Developing an integrated case management approach

For the purposes of management and planning, the rehabilitative process can be divided into five phases as depicted in Figure 7.1.

This type of overview would be introduced to the new clients when they first present at the clinic for implant consideration. This overview would be used to enable the clients to develop an understanding of what is involved in the overall process of rehabilitation and to work to temper expectations that may relate to the technology as a *quick fix* for their hearing and listening problems.

Depending on the model of intervention presently used within an implant clinic, existing clients may well lie at various points along this continuum. For newer clients not yet implanted, it is feasible that they will have undergone a number of medical and audiological assessments by the time the need for more in-depth counselling and discussion about their suitability as candidates arises. This would mean, on the one hand, that the client and the clinician have been developing a rapport, and that the

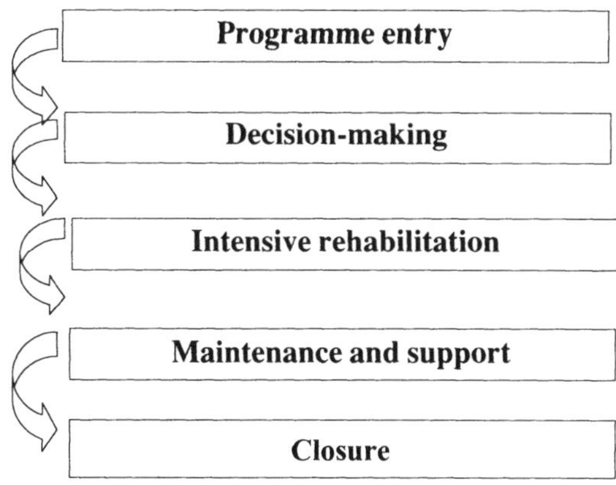

Figure 7.1: Five phases of rehabilitation.

clinician has been developing a mental picture about the client's needs and disposition. In addition, the clients' expectations about their likelihood of being implanted have probably been steadily rising as they see themselves *successfully* moving through various stages of the assessment process. And not without good reason. If prospective candidates are told by differing clinicians or surgeons that they have passed this or that test, or that they are medically *suitable*, it is quite reasonable for them to expect to proceed to implantation. This is well and good if no problems arise. However, if and when problems arise, the clinic and clients find themselves in a situation of potential conflict, that requires careful management. The implementation of an integrated staged or *case management approach* – centred on the five phases of the rehabilitative process – may serve to minimize or eliminate many of the problems already noted.

Principles of the case management approach

The idea behind a client-centred approach is that the prospective candidate would move through a series of interviews, assessments and skill development programmes with a view to coming to an informed decision about cochlear implantation. Several factors are considered to be central to ensuring the success of this approach:

- Clients receive a clear overview, in writing or graphical form, of the assessment and decision-making process.
- The client's partners or significant others should be involved in the process wherever practicable.

- Clients should be informed, up front, that the decision to implant is based upon the integration of information taken from all aspects of the assessment and preparation process. In consequence, they will not receive feedback concerning success or failure, at the completion of a particular assessment (e.g. promontory stimulation).
- The assessments should be scheduled to occur in a timely fashion so that the process is not dragged out nor the clients unduly stressed by the decision-making process.
- The decision to implant is taken as a team, with all aspects of the decision-making process being given adequate weighting in the decision-making process.

For informed consent to be achieved, it is essential that clients enter the rehabilitation process, properly informed and prepared for the decisions confronting them. This process may easily be biased for both clients and colleagues, if one member of the assessment team gives the client an indication that implantation can proceed, when the others have yet to have their input. Surgical readiness, for example, forms only one part of the assessment process. The assessment and decision-making phase is concerned with developing, in conjunction with the client, a programme of interventions that will best address the client's overall rehabilitation need. It is premature to proceed to implantation until the broader audiological and psychosocial rehabilitative issues have been given adequate consideration and weighting within the decision-making process. For example, the recently deafened child of a family of signing and culturally Deaf people may be audiologically suitable for implantation, but in every other sense – not suitable at all.

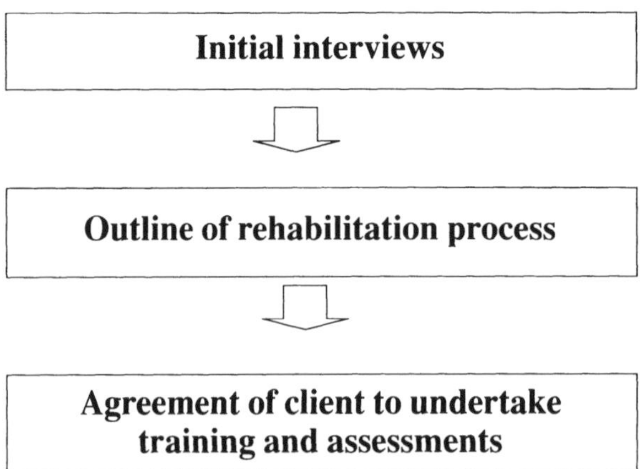

Figure 7.2: Programme entry.

Programme entry

For many Deafened people there is no clear point in time when they can say that they became totally deaf. For many, the onset of deafness was experienced as slow transition into deafness, as the disease process proceeded along its varying and unpredictable course. Unlike those whose onset was acute and rapid (e.g. from a head injury like Jeff, resulting in total deafness), the point at which the person with a progressive loss becomes officially *deafened* is uncertain. Similarly, the point at which the person moves from being hearing-impaired or deafened to officially becoming an *implant candidate* is also blurry. An observer could be forgiven for thinking that all Deafened people are considered to be candidates until a decision is made not to implant them. This problem is underscored by the fact that clinics tend to only offer an implant *programme*, rather than seeing themselves as centres of hearing rehabilitation. From the client's perspective, the transition period from Deafened person to implant candidate can be likened to treading water endlessly, until a person in a nearby boat finally decides to throw you a line, by offering implantation. Yet the fact of the matter is that all the while you could have swum to a nearby pontoon and gained assistance in living with deafness.

Given that many clients may:

- wander in the borderland of not quite being deaf enough for quite some time;
- have to wait for an implant because of a shortage in resources;
- never be implanted;

it becomes critical from the outset to communicate clearly with new clients about the type of service being offered, the processes involved and the range of outcomes that might be achieved. The first point of intervention therefore, is not some sort of medical or audiological assessment, but the initial interview, which serves as a gateway into the decision-making process.

The initial interview: engaging the client in a rehabilitative relationship

Prior to commencing any form of assessment, the case manager (i.e the clinician responsible for coordinating the client's rehabilitation programme) conducts an initial, *scoping* interview with the new client. Ideally, this interview would be conducted in conjunction with the team's psychologist, social worker or rehabilitation counsellor. As the name suggests, a scoping interview consists of a series of broad, open-ended questions, that are concerned with developing a picture of the client's experience of deafness, its impact in their life and their initial motivations for seeking implantation. Questions that might be asked during this initial interview are:

- To begin today, would you mind telling me about what happened to your hearing?
- What would you say have been the greatest consequences, for you, of losing your hearing (prompt questions may follow concerning relationships, employment, social activities, stress and health)?
- What services have you already used?
- What did you find un/helpful about these services?
- How do you think cochlear implantation might help you?

The same questions may also be addressed to the spouse, whose quality of life has also been affected by the loss of hearing. These types of questions, supported with supplementary and exploratory questions, should result in an interview that extends for 45 minutes to an hour. At the end of this interview, one ought to be able to develop a story about the client's experience of onset, not dissimilar to that presented in Chapter 2. At the end of this interview, the clinician should have a good idea about the types of concerns the client has (e.g. relational, education, employment, social, health concerns) and the range of issues that may need to be encompassed within their rehabilitation programme.

Decision-making

It is at this time that an overview of the clinic's services can be introduced, in terms of the phases discussed above and with regard to the various components of otological and audiological assessments. Once the programme overview has been covered, the client may be invited to become actively involved in the programme by becoming an informed decision-maker. This entails:

- participation in the development of communication skills in a group setting;
- getting to know other Deafened people, including people with a *range* of experiences with and without the cochlear implant;
- learning to adjust to deafness, through interaction and self-education;
- participating in various clinical assessments normally associated with pre-implantation.

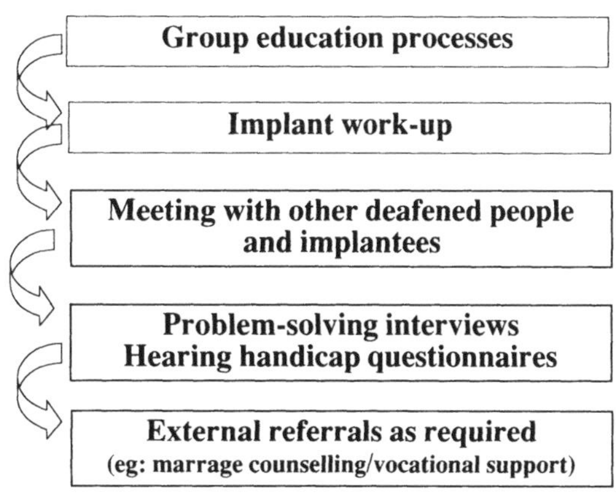

Figure 7.3: Decision-making.

These steps (summarized in Figure 7.3) are included in the process for several reasons. First, a decision about remaking oneself as a Deafened person needs to be understood as something that one logically works towards – it is not a whim or an impulse. Second, in the foreseeable future, the majority of clients who receive a cochlear implant will retain a degree of hearing disability and therefore require assertiveness and communication skills. Third, with adventitious loss, there has been an experience of trauma and personal upheaval (and as we have seen possibly including loss of job or life partner) that needs to be recognized, validated and resolved. Fourth, unrealistic expectations need to be tempered. Finally, a working relationship needs to developed with the clients and their partners, that can be sustained through the long and often tedious process of rehabilitation that lies ahead. In the event that the clinic is unable to offer the client implantation, interventions may be continued with a view to developing alternative communication skills. For those clients implanted, the working relationship can be developed with a view to enabling clients to pace themselves through the adjustment process, and to maximize their communication skills and social confidence through the use of appropriate communication strategies and assertiveness skills.

At this point clients have engaged in the process of remaking themselves. It is a process concerned as much with the development of personal identity as it is with communication skills. Identity is something developed in relation to others – such as via a peer group. The purpose of the rehabilitative process is not to deny one's disability by trying to stamp it out with a technology, but to enable the clients to integrate their past experiences of disability and communication, with a new way of living that encompasses the management of technology, communication strategies, others and the self, into the social process we call social interaction.

Contracting with your clients: identifying rehabilitative goals and problematic issues

Following the initial interview and participation in a group-based skills development programme, and amidst the audiological and medical assessments, it is timely to have the client and partner complete a hearing handicap questionnaire as an aid to identifying personal issues critical to the progress of the rehablitative intervention. The Code-Müller Protocols (discussed in Chapter 6) may also be completed at this time and used for counselling clients concerning their expectations of benefit arising from the intervention. Assessments relating to the physical suitability for an implant or a hearing aid follow a technical rationality that is driven by the technology. The nature of client/clinician interactions within these settings is dictated to a large extent by the assessment protocols associated with the technologies of interest. A separate session is required for assessments associated with psychosocial disposition. These new interactions provide the clinician with a further opportunity to identify issues that may not have arisen previously but which may be important in developing a programme of rehabilitation addressing the many concerns held by clients and partners. There are a number of good hearing handicap questionnaires available that can be used for this purpose. Ideally, the one chosen should not be too long (e.g. less than 50 items) and be suitable for scoring so that pre- and post-measures of intervention may be obtained. The questionnaire should also come in a format that can be completed by the partner and by the clinician. Alternatively, it should be adaptable for use with partners and clinicians.

Coupled with the technological assessments, the results of the scoping interview and personal disposition questionnaires (hearing handicap and expectations), the clinician managing the assessment process has a large amount of information about the client, the nature of treatments that may be of benefit and so on. While the activities involved in the treatment plan and the requirements for the client may be, from your perspective, routine and quite apparent, they may not be so clear from the client's perspective. As the noted counselling adviser Gerald Egan (1975: 24) observed, 'many therapists fail to tell their clients much about the therapeutic process ... clients are often expected to buy a pig-in-a-poke without much assurance that it will turn out to be very succulent pork'. Egan continues to point out that while the contracting process should not be overwhelming for the client, it does need to make apparent the clinic's expectations for the client. Certainly, clinics routinely take certain steps to ensure that individuals consent to surgery and its associated risks.

Contracting takes this process a step further by ensuring that the client is aware or prepared for the array of post-implant interventions that are required. This is particularly important as many clinics in the past have adopted a ***wait and see*** approach to rehabilitation, indicating that only those clients who have a poor communication outcome require rehabilitation. As such, rehabilitation is associated with failure and clients are not well motivated to engage in the therapy required to achieve the results desired. A rehabilitation contract serves to circumvent these problems.

A rehabilitation contract between a clinic and a client is achieved through a process of counselling and negotiation, such as that associated with the Code-Müller Protocols. Following the negotiation process, agreement is reached concerning the range of treatments and activities that will make up the person's individual rehabilitation programme. Depending on the clients' disposition and motivation, pre-implant interventions such as communication training may be prescribed as a strategy for settling them into the helping process and for calibrating their attitudes towards the type of behaviours they will need to use following implantation. Post-implant therapies such as auditory training should also be planned into the contract. In the happy event that the clients move rapidly through the programme then they can move on quickly. But as can be envisaged, it is much easier to say to clients that they have progressed through the programme quickly than to say the opposite.

Intensive rehabilitation

During this phase, the rehabilitation programme proper is implemented. Where implantation is concerned, Figure 7.5 provides an overview of the steps involved.

Beyond implantation

Following implantation, the client-centred approach to counselling becomes especially important. For many, the months following switch-on (or hook-up) are something akin to a roller-coaster ride, as clients work to make sense of the auditory input they now receive. As auditory input becomes increasingly useful, clients will have differing expectations concerning the directions they want to go in and about the rate of their progress. Comparative measures for the experience of hearing handicap and optimism about the future are very useful for tempering these types of expectations. It is important for people to know that it is normal to feel

Client's name: ______________________________

Partner's name: ______________________________

Programme aim: To enhance (insert name) communication and listening skills

Programme objectives: At the end of this rehabilitation programme (client's name) will have:

i) learnt new skills for managing difficult communication settings
ii) developed assertiveness skills
iii) received a cochlear implant

Client responsibilities: (insert name) undertakes to:

i) attend the clinic, on a fortnightly basis, for individual communication training (with partner present) prior to implantation;
ii) practise prescribed exercises at home and maintain log;
iii) undergo cochlear implantation ;
iv) attend an intensive post-implant group training programme consisting of a) three 2-hour sessions in the first week post hook-up; b) two 2-hour sessions in the second week post hook-up; c) one 2-hour session in the third and fourth weeks post hook-up; at least three additional 1-hour sessions as then required
v) participate in a group-based training programme 3 months post switch-on.

The plan will be reviewed six months from today: ________________(review date).

Signed: ______________________ (client) date : ______________
Signed: ______________________ (partner) date : ______________
Signed: ______________________ (audiologist) date : ______________

Figure 7.4a: Rehabilitation plan.

Client's name: ______________________________

Partner's name: ______________________________

Programme aim: ______________________________

____

____

Programme objectives: ______________________________

____

____

Expected outcomes: ______________________________

____

____

Client responsibilities: ______________________________

____

____

____

Signed: ______________ (client) date : ______________
Signed: ______________ (partner) date : ______________
Signed: ______________ (audiologist) date : ______________

Figure 7.4b: Rehabilitation plan.

- **Audiology**
  - Surgical debriefing
  - Switch-on programming assessments
  - Periodic mapping and assessments
  - Individual communication therapies
- **Psychosocial**
  - Counselling re: expectations
  - Periodic psychosocial assessment
  - Group skills programme
  - External referrals as indicated
  - Peer support

Figure 7.5: Intensive rehabilitation.

very up or rather down at particular points in the rehabilitation process. It is also helpful to be able to point out to people when their affect is outside the norms of usual experience. But of greatest importance is recognizing where the clients are at as compared with where they want to be, given where the clinician thinks they are likely to end up.

Once again, the CMP can be used as a counselling strategy here. Managing this part of the process is the real work of setting the direction of post-implant training and support, and for working towards closure of the intensive period of support that has accompanied implantation. This process will be different every time, depending on the client's auditory benefit, age, sex, and life stage, not to mention their personal hopes and aspirations. Coupled with this will be the need to monitor and manage the partner's personal needs now that so much as changed in their lives, yet again.

As clients' communication skills improve and they become more socially independent, they may engage in more social activities than they did previously. These activities may need to be supported with group-based communication training and confidence building, so that clients may become quite adept in their new environments. Similarly, some clients may wish to think about returning to employment, or undertaking further training. This means that clinicians may need to organize referrals to an appropriate employment service. As part of establishing a holistic rehabilitation service, clinics should have a referral mechanism in place that ensures clients can make a smooth transition between hearing and vocational rehabilitation services. Figure 7.6 provides an overview of what such a structure might look like. As can be seen, it is a dynamic model, requiring interaction between the implant clinic and the vocational rehabilitation provider. Given the rehabilitation needs of existing deafened adults and the nature of the labour market, it is reasonable to expect that vocational rehabilitation may take some time to achieve and that some clients will not return to paid work.

As the mutually identified therapeutic goals have been addressed, it comes time to develop a plan, in conjunction with the client, to bring the intensive phase of the intervention to a close and to re-establish the client at Phase 4 of the programme – ongoing support. This involves a momentary return to the decision-making process, involving a discussion of the client's hopes and aspirations, tempered in the light of what a clinic can be realistically expected to provide. Thus part of such discussions involves enabling the client to recognize that the time is approaching for them to begin to move on and that the clinic's role in their life will gradually diminish.

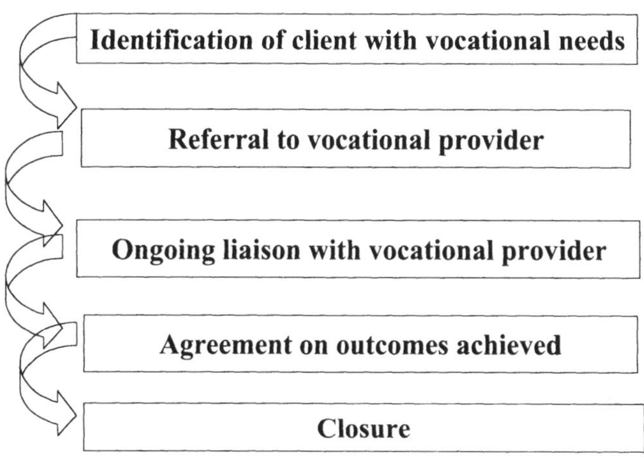

Figure 7.6: Vocational rehabilitation.

Ongoing support

Phase 4 is concerned with ongoing support of the implantee and their family. The programme of intervention might encompass a range of activities, depending on the needs of the clients and available clinical resources. Practically, this may entail a group-based follow-up, initially every three months, tapering off over time to once a year or as required. In addition, clients may feel the need simply to come in for a periodic chat.

The maintenance phase fulfils several key psychosocial functions. First, it provides clients with a structured process of support as they make the transition to being independent hearing people. Without a clear rite of passage, a sense of awkwardness may develop between the clients and the

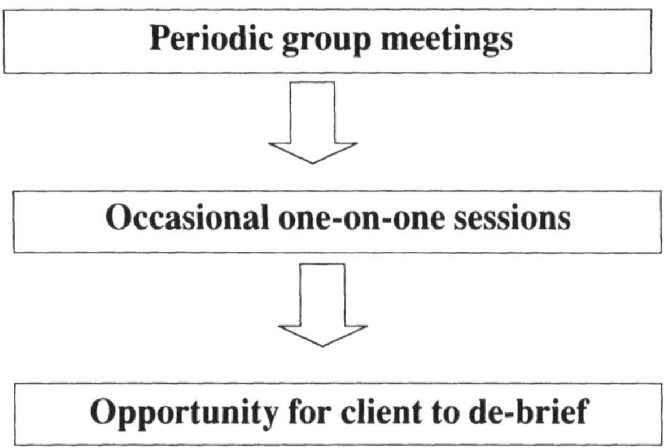

Figure 7.7: Ongoing support.

clinician. The clinician feels that he or she has done all or as much as they can for the clients and that it is time for the clients to move on. Yet through the intensive process of rehabilitation, the clients have become quite emotionally bonded to the clinician. This is not a bond that can simply be severed. It needs to be released gently. Without careful management, the clients may *drop out* of the service, simply because they are not sure what to do or when it is appropriate for them to visit the clinic. Alternatively, apparent *problems* with the map may arise as the clients seek a legitimate reason to come in for support. *Chat time* then needs to be seen as a central part of clients' follow-up and support programmes and needs to be planned for, rather than squeezed on to the end of a mapping session.

Indeed, visits to the clinic serve as an emotional release valve for clients. The visit provides an opportunity for them to *sound-off* about the difficulties they may have been experiencing with the device, family members, work mates or friends. It may also be that when they are with their clinician, clients feel that this is the one place where their needs are really understood and where they are really accepted, so visiting the clinic becomes a relaxing experience.

As clients have progressed through their rehabilitation programme, many of the day-to-day difficulties of living with deafness and an implant should have begun to settle down. As one approaches closure of the rehabilitation side of the intervention, the clients will have become settled into the rhythm of their new life, complete with its inherent imperfections. As part of the settling process, the clients' need to sound-off or draw emotional support will lessen. At the same time, it becomes important to teach the clients alternative ways of releasing pent up emotion. Some of these may be covered in group sessions and address issues such as stress management and relaxation. But at this stage it may be timely to introduce the clients to the idea of keeping a journal of experiences, both positive and negative. A summary of the log may serve as a way of keeping the clinician up-to-date with events that occur in the intervening months between follow-up sessions. At a deeper level, the log will provide clients with a mechanism for identifying the issues that set them off so that they can then learn to deal with them more effectively. Logs also serve as way of letting go of the emotions associated with such activities.

Maintenance and closure

At this point in the clients' rehabilitation programme, it comes time to prepare them for closure. In preparing for closure one would conduct a review interview. Within the review interview, progress made with the clients during their rehabilitation programme to date would be noted, with particular emphasis being placed on the various milestones achieved (e.g. 41 per cent increase in hearing sensitivity; 34 per cent increase in quality of life; 28 per cent increase in self-esteem, successful employment placement; 50 per cent increase in weekly income; adoption of two new hobbies; 35 per cent reduction in stress). Moreover, the opportunity may be taken to review those goals that were not achieved and to discuss with the clients, what, if anything, can be done to address them. Where further work needs to be undertaken, the clinician should contract accordingly. Otherwise it comes time to acknowledge all the work the clients have done and what they have achieved in remaking themselves as one who uses a cochlear implant effectively.

Closure entails a rite of passage that denotes a change in the nature of the relationship between the clients and the clinic. It is a time for recognizing the process that has been undertaken, and the outcomes achieved. Figure 7.8 provides an overview of this process in its entirety. In preparation for closure the clinician has been gradually introducing the clients to other support mechanisms so that when the rehabilitation programme is complete, they will not feel cast aside. Clinic-centred mechanisms (such as the occasional morning tea or barbecue) might be put in place that provide an opportunity for clients to maintain contact with the clinic if they wish to do so. The nature of the rite of passage is not as important as the event itself. For some it might simply entail a final interview, with the clinician and client conducting a review, identifying on-going sources of support and contact, and concluding with a handshake. Others might prefer a graduation ceremony or simply to go out and party!! The important thing is for clients to realize that sameness (as discussed in Chapter 3) as been achieved, that life has resumed a degree of normality for us and that the intensive work of personal reformation now yields to the day-to-day effort of getting on with life.

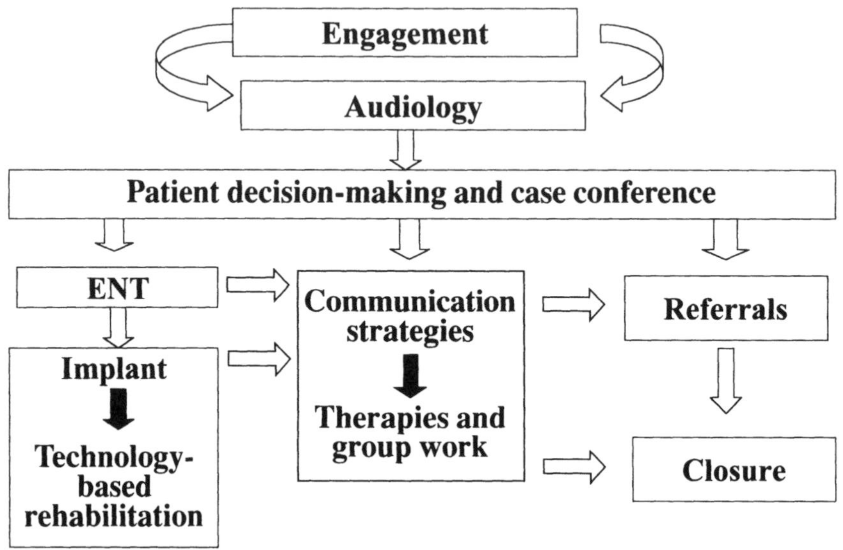

Figure 7.8: Rehabilitation overview.

Chapter 8

Enhancing employment outcomes

Anthony Hogan, Lee Kethel, Kate White and Andrea Lynch

Introduction

Employment has been a key issue facing people with hearing loss for well over a century. Indeed, much of the push towards deaf education that originated in the nineteenth century was concerned to ensure that deaf people were able to take their places as equals within the broader community (Winzer, 1993). Historically little attention has been given to the social needs of adults with hearing loss who do not identify with the Deaf community. These people, like people within the Deaf community, comprise a socioeconomically disadvantaged group within the community. Wilson et al. (1999) have demonstrated that Deafened people in particular have considerably poorer health than other Australians. In addition, Deafened people are 1.5 times more likely than other Australians to be unemployed (Hogan, Taylor and Code, 1999), and many live on low incomes (Taylor et al., 1999).

Despite these poor outcomes, advances in rehabilitative interventions, such as the cochlear implant, have resulted in implantees being 2–3 times more likely to be employed than non-implantees (Hogan et al., 1999). Elsewhere, in the large United Kingdom implant study (Summerfield and Marshall, 1995) the receipt of a cochlear implant was not found to improve a client's employment situation per se. Overall, it is unclear whether those seeking implants had a better rate of employment prior to deafness than those without implants or whether the implant process actually results in improved employment prospects for the recipient. Certainly, interview materials recorded with implantees indicate that the cochlear implant results in improved social relations in the workplace (Hogan, 1997). However, while enhanced hearing sensitivity may assist an individual in obtaining employment, it will not in itself result in a spontaneous improvement in the individual's overall employment skills. At best, one may expect the implantees to remain in their pre-implant field of employment and progress along their career path in the usual fashion or that they would undergo some form of employment preparation (re)training programme. Over time, several outcomes should occur.

First, it could be expected that a larger proportion of implantees would obtain or retain paid employment and that their workforce participation rate would remain comparable with that of the population and increase towards the population norm. The data presented in Chapter 2, for example, showed that presently the workforce participation rate for implantees was 56.3 per cent compared with a population rate of 67.4 per cent. This rate varies considerably depending on the age of those concerned. For example, of those aged less than 55 years, the participation rate was 76.8 per cent compared with a population rate of 78.6 per cent. Second, the proportion of people earning equal to and/or greater than average weekly earnings should improve. Indeed, as was noted in Chapter 2, income, rather than employment, is the major issue facing Deafened people. As such, it may not be employment but rather access to promotion that is the key issue to monitor with regards to the longer-term economic benefits of implants for Deafened people.

Overall then, access to and success within employment remain key issues for Deafened people. Indeed, as many people considering cochlear implantation cite return to work, or the maintenance of their existing employment, as a key goal within their hearing rehabilitation programme, it is critical that these matters be taken into account.

It is important then that implant clinics take appropriate steps to ensure that every opportunity is taken to enhance employment opportunities for their clients. However, as vocational services are not a core aspect of cochlear implant programmes, an effective and efficient referral pathway between the implant clinic and a vocational service provider is required. While there are a large number of vocational and employment service providers available in the community, the preferred vocational provider needs the following qualities:

1. to have a broad network of service centres;
2. to employ rehabilitation staff within the clinic's catchment area, who have expertise in working with Deafened clients;
3. to be able to provide a case manager who would act as a pivot person to liaise between the implant clinic and the various providers across the state.

The case manager's role is to act as an interface between the clinic and the various services it offers across the target area. The case manager accepts referrals from the clinic and organizes their distribution to staff located regionally. The case manager in turn, follows up the progress of respective clients and reports back to the clinic at case conferences which are held periodically. Figure 7.6 (see p. 127) depicts the referral process for vocational care of implantees.

With the assistance of vocational rehabilitation service providers, clinics can ensure that clients access the range of additional support services they require, without placing additional strain on their own resources.

Enhancing employment outcomes: a worked example at the Mater Adult Cochlear Implant Programme Brisbane

Staff employed at the Mater Adult Cochlear Implant Programme Brisbane identified employment as a key concern for their clients. With this in mind, CRS Australia (a national vocational rehabilitation service provider for people with disabilities) in Queensland was approached for assistance through a local case manager (a speech pathologist who had extensive experience working with deafened clients in a vocational setting) and the referral mechanism was established. The case manager's role was to act as an interface between the clinic and the various vocational rehabilitation support services offered by CRS Australia across the target area. The case manager accepted referrals from the clinic and organized their distribution to professional employment services staff located regionally. The case manager, in turn, followed up the progress of respective clients and reported back at case conferences which were held periodically.

Eighteen clients were invited by clinic staff to participate in the programme; 11 clients indicated their willingness to participate and they were referred to CRS Australia for assistance. Clients have differing vocational needs that will vary depending upon their age and experience of deafness. These factors include:

- duration of deafness;
- time of onset (with regards to education and employment skills);
- present qualifications and work experience;
- current communication skills (including telephone skills);
- presence of other disabilities.

Table 8.1 provides an overview of the 11 clients who participated in the employment study. It can be seen that seven of the respondents had post-school education, while three of the 11 participants had at least one

Table 8.1: Demographic overview of participants in employment study

ID	AGE	SEX	EDUCATION	DISABILITY	YRS OF DEAFNESS	PREVIOUS EMPLOYMENT
1	21	F	University	Ill health	15–20	Student
2	53	F	Grade 10	Nil	15–20	Office work/mother
3	49	F	TAFE[1]	Nil	>25	Office work/mother
4	22	M	Grade 10/TAFE	Psychiatric disability	22	Student
5	51	M	Primary	Nil	<5	Police officer
6	32	F	TAFE	Nil	32	
7	43	M	TAFE	Multiple disabilities	<5	
8	44	M	TAFE	Nil	10–15	Electrician
9	44	F	TAFE	Nil	>25	Draftsman/mother
10	35	M	High school	Nil	10–15	Technician
11	40	F	Grade 10	Nil	40	Cleaner/kitchen hand

[1]TAFE (Technical and Further Education) is a government-based training institution, similar to a polytechnic in the United Kingdom, that provides trade and similar vocational training programmes.

additional disability. Most respondents had some previous work experience in trade, clerical or unskilled positions. Their average age was 39.5 years.

Table 8.2 provides data on the employment outcomes from the pilot project. Three respondents achieved an employment outcome although one subsequently withdrew as a result of ill health (cancer). A further four respondents enrolled in various employment retraining and employment-related training programmes. The remaining four withdrew due to personal difficulties and/or family responsibilities.

Table 8.2: Employment outcomes from the study

SUBJECT	OUTCOME
1	Obtained casual work following intervention; presently unable to work due to ill health (cancer).
2	Withdrew from vocational programme: family illness.
3	Accepted into rehabilitation programme. Elected to transfer to supported employment agency. Currently part-time work and full-time university study.
4	Assessed for vocationally-based rehabilitation programme but did not proceed as studying full-time with support.
5	Completed vocational rehabilitation programme with part-time work outcome.
6	Withdrew due to pregnancy.
7	Accepted for vocational rehabilitation programme, withdrew due to difficulties with multiple disabilities.
8	Accepted for vocational rehabilitation programme. Did not complete programme due to difficulties. Currently self-employed.
9	Withdrew due to marital separation and desire to undertake full-time studies. Currently studying full-time.
10	Assessed for vocational rehabilitation programme but did not proceed as studying full-time with support. Currently has part-time work.
11	Currently working (not eligible for access to vocational rehabilitation programme).

Overall, it can be seen that participants in the pilot programme had a high level of post-school training when compared with the overall sample of Deafened people examined in Chapter 2. The employment referral procedure, established between the implant clinic and a vocational rehabilitation provider, resulted in 7 of the 11 participants obtaining an improved employment outcome within a relatively short period of time (6–8 months). However, a range of factors, other than deafness, impacted on the likelihood of the remaining clients achieving an employment outcome. The first of these is the demography of the group itself. A middle-aged person, with few transferable skills and limited employment experience, with one or more disabilities, is considered to be a difficult person to place in employment. Second, the presence of an additional disease process or other disability (e.g. a head injury) resulted in clients being unable to complete their vocational rehabilitation programme or return to work. Third, everyday life events, such as having a baby or being required to care for a sick relative, also impacted on participants.

Historically, people with hearing loss have faced difficulties both obtaining and retaining paid employment. The data reported in Chapter 2 indicate that the workforce participation rate of clients is presently 9–11 per cent below the population average. The employment referral process reported here indicates that this gap may be reduced through the provision of vocational rehabilitation services in conjunction with cochlear implantation. The actual contribution of cochlear implants to employment opportunities for Deafened people remains unclear and requires continuing examination within a prospective study.

Realistic expectations need to be held with regard to the level of impact an implant programme can have on clients' vocational prospects. Certainly, it would be expected that clients in paid employment prior to implantation would maintain their pre-implant vocational status and continue to progress in their employment following implantation. Of course, there are career barriers facing Deafened people and this needs to be recognized as it will be a problem for some time to come. In cases where clients have recently withdrawn from their occupation due to hearing problems, it would be hoped that they would return to such employment following implantation. In cases where the clients have withdrawn from their vocation for a long time prior to implantation, it is likely that a process of vocational reskilling will be required before those people will return to the workforce.

It was noted that average weekly earnings for implantees are presently well below those of the rest of the population and that this may result, in part, to barriers to advancement in the workplace. Given the historic and educational factors that have led to this situation, it will be more difficult to improve this outcome for Deafened people quickly. Nonetheless, changes in average weekly earnings may be brought about routinely as newly Deafened adults directly enter the implant programme, therein avoiding some of the economic problems associated with loss of employment and/or early retirement due to deafness. Second, by enhancing the rate of employment (and therefore incomes) among longer-term Deafened people, as demonstrated in this chapter, the rate may also increase. Third, in conjunction with affirmative action policies administered by governments, as representative numbers of people with disabilities come to be employed in more senior positions the rate may also rise.

Enhancing workplace outcomes

Integral to enabling deafened adults to access retraining and employment is the need to address communication in the workplace. Working in collaboration with vocational rehabilitation providers, clinics may support implantees in the workplace by ensuring that inclusive communication strategies are taught to co-workers. These programmes are usually workshop-based and are designed to sensitize co-workers to the communication needs of Deafened adults. Programme topics might include participants undergoing an unfair hearing test and a lip-reading test. Unfair hearing tests are commercially available, but can also be made in your own clinic. An unfair hearing test may be constructed by recording a word list and having it passed through frequency-based filters so that key high or low frequency sounds are lost from the sounds presented. Participants are required to write down the words they think they have heard. Responses are then workshopped, highlighting the difficulties of hearing in background noise, the similarity of words and the nature of mistakes made. Various lip-reading tests can also be administered and the workshop approach repeated.

The key to these presentations is to keep them lively, emphasizing the learning goals and avoiding getting bogged down in dreary technical details. The aim of the intervention is to highlight the communication difficulties confronting people with impaired hearing in a workplace culture that centres on a conversation-based culture and then to valorize the use of those well-known communication strategies such as facing the person, speaking slowly and clearly, having the person's attention before commencing a statement, managing light and so on.

Conclusion

Finding or retaining paid employment is an important rehabilitative goal for people with cochlear implants. While taking into account a variety of historical difficulties, employment outcomes for people with cochlear implants appear to be improving, despite the likely presence of a glass ceiling that may prevent career advancement for skilled individuals. Structural employment problems such as age, the absence of transferable work skills and the presence of additional disease processes or disabilities, may be barriers to employment outcomes for specific clients. In such instances, the systematic provision of vocational services as part of the client's rehabilitation programme may serve to enhance employment outcomes. For the newly Deafened adult, vocational assistance may be provided to protect the person's existing employment and to ensure a smooth transition from rehabilitation back to work. Taking these factors into account, workforce participation and average weekly earnings better reflect the socioeconomic benefits of cochlear implantation than crude reported improvements in employment status.

CHAPTER 9

The everyday benefits of cochlear implantation

Introduction

This chapter begins with an overview of the perceived benefits of cochlear implantation from the implantees' perspective.

A narrative on benefits

Successful implantation of an appropriate cochlear prosthesis enhances a Deafened person's ability to interact with people within the various communication environments that make up everyday life. For people who choose an implant, the device represents a commonsense step taken in response to the onset of deafness:

> What made you decide to ... have an implant?
> Basically, I just couldn't see a good reason not to.[Laughter] (Jean)

> What led you to decide to have the implant?
> Because I couldn't hear [Laughs]
> Would you do it again?
> Of course! ... It's made an immeasurable difference (Gena).

For Gena, implantation meant that her life was back on track again; she could live out being a wife, a mum, a grandmother, a friend and a professional as she knew how it should be lived out. No, life is not easy. Communication remains imperfect, but it is far nearer to being normal than it ever was. For Gena and implantees generally, the benefits of implantation can be understood in terms of social connectedness and an enhanced ability to communicate.

Social connectedness

Cochlear implantation enables recipients to hear environmental sounds. This outcome enables the individual to participate in daily activities widely regarded as normal. These activities include being able to hear and respond to the telephone or doorbell ringing, through to being able to share the pleasure of country sounds and bird calls with a loved one. The first set of these experiences is functional, enabling the recipient to get on with daily activities without having constantly to worry that one has missed a call or a visitor. The second set of these experiences enables the recipient to share in the subtle pleasures of life that 'hearing people' take for granted:

> Well, the advantages of the sounds you can hear. You can hear bird sounds and I mean, even environmental sounds and things like footsteps walking and cars going past. Water moving. All these environmental sounds tend to make you feel that you're in a living place, not a dead place. (Gena)

Implantation is about being normal again, where being normal means that one does not have to think constantly about being deaf. As Liz has so succinctly observed, 'I feel more whole. [I] don't feel sort of as though I'm a freak. As though I'm just like the same as everyone else.' Implantation enables the Deafened person to pass without seeming to contest the taken-for-granted rules of everyday interaction. Implantation reduces the socially isolating effects of hearing loss and removes or reduces the individual's sense of being a social burden. For many Deafened adults, the onset of hearing loss was experienced so slowly that they had forgotten just how much they used to hear. Implantation means the restoration of the ability to participate in the everyday world in unexceptional ways: 'those little touches that keep you in touch with the world' (Rick). Implantation is regarded as a transforming *medium* that enables recipients to resume life as they want to live it, just as Gena described it.

Enhanced ability to communicate

One of the most extensive benefits of cochlear implantation reported by recipients is within the domain of family and social communication. Implantation reduces communication problems experienced within the family. This outcome is reported with regard to both the quality and quantity of communication. Gena, for example, used sign language to communicate with her family. However, she felt that she just missed out on too much of the everyday communication required to nurture loving and effective relationships and broader personal networks. Gena reported that following implantation she was able to participate in conversations that got right down to the nitty-gritty of everyday interactions, rather than being left to vagaries of only receiving information in so-called 'vital' communications. Having once heard, the alternative world of signing deafness is not considered as a viable alternative, but seen as limited in terms of access to communication and the social:

> Having been completely deaf, I know how much I missed out on at that time ... And how much different it is now that I'm back into the hearing world again. Even though it's not perfect now! It's still is such an enormous improvement. (Gena)

Cochlear implantation reduces the extent to which communication problems are experienced within day-to-day communication. Partners do not have to work as hard to make themselves understood. There is less need for repetition of statements and increased opportunity for intimacy. At work, co-workers do not have to try as hard to make themselves understood and external support resources, such as signing interpreters, are not required. At the broader level, implantation enables one to resume social activities as they used to be lived. Fiona reflects on the extent of such changes:

> [my partner] loves visiting and chatting to people, and going and mixing. And I wouldn't before. I'd just stop home. But now, we go out a lot and mix with people. And of course we've got the family and yeah ... it is different.

Implantees report being able to talk to family members on the telephone. This outcome also encompasses some respondents who may be regarded as 'poor' performers who are able to conduct somewhat structured conversations with family members they know well.

Implantation may result in an enhancement of the implantee's social confidence and independence, resulting mainly from a reduction in social anxiety. Implantees can carry on a conversation in circumstances where they previously would have withdrawn from social participation:

> not very long after I got this ... I was up there [in the bank] and this man came walking towards me. Now if someone came towards me to ask me something before, I'd just say I'm sorry I'm deaf I can't help you. Only after I had this one. But with this one, I could see him coming. He came up and asked me where the club was. I never hesitated. I knew where it was and I told him. That's the only time it's happened since I've had this one; but if someone came up to me now it wouldn't worry me. (Liz)

Becoming confident, being able to leave the deaf world behind means becoming a new person, no longer afraid to 'barge' up to people and to start a conversation (Fiona). Simply knowing that one is able to do the little things enhances the implantee's confidence for everyday activities. Prior to implantation, simple requests for directions proved to be times of stress and hassle. Now they are managed with greater ease and confidence. For Liz, it almost seems like fun, like 'go on – do it again! Help me appreciate how well I'm doing now!' The implant also provides less tangible but important benefits:

> [I have] more confidence [pause] and probably a feeling of well-being and self-esteem had probably come back. The feeling I won't be put down. But I'm OK, but so are you, type of thing, you know, that sort of thing. (Carol)

Implantation means being able to get on with the everyday activities that hearing people enjoy:

> I was crocheting and the theme song, you might say it's *Home and Away* [came on the TV]. I can look down and crochet like that and I can hear the sound. I know when they're singing ... what part of it...I wouldn't be without it, not for anything. (Fiona)

Implantation makes it easier to hear the children speak, to distinguish people's voices from each other and communicate without having constantly to watch faces. However, following implantation Deafened people still have to struggle with everyday communication problems like trying to listen to lectures from bearded university professors. Communication in group settings remains difficult. Implantation can mean the opportunity to make up for the many life opportunities lost because of deafness: 'I don't want to waste any more time' (Carol). 'Getting on with it' means that implantees can take up positions of responsibility or challenges previously denied Deafened people such as being the secretary of their local club, participating in meetings and taking minutes. For a long time, the sound of implants has been referred to like hearing 'Donald Duck talking under water' (*Daily Telegraph*, 1987). Newer speech processors have taken the implant beyond the problems of early times: 'I'm actually picking up the sound of your voice. Things like that, it really makes my day' (Carol).

Not all the benefits of implantation necessarily result in pleasure; some are painful. A number of respondents report experiencing people differently. Auditory input coupled with lip-reading means that it is possible to notice aspects of people's personalities that had previously gone unchecked. Some people, previously regarded as friendly, have been found to speak in either patronizing or sarcastic tones. People once thought friendly appear to be unpleasant or at least have unpleasant aspects to their personalities. Conversely, help needed to undertake everyday activities is no longer required. The helper posing as friend moves on to find someone else to 'look after'. These experiences add depth and richness to relationships even if some relationships have to be reworked. Implantation provides one with the opportunity to grow as a person and make more informed judgements about people involved in one's personal network.

Work

The benefit of implantation at the work level is that people are likely to be treated more favourably. Because people are more able to hear and speak, others will think that they are more competent and treat them accordingly. In turn, they may retain employment and possibly even gain a promotion. A partner observes:

> I think the implant has made a big difference to him in terms of his work. Um, it's, often it's not so much what a person is able to do in a job as what others perceive him as being able to do so, that even though his ability hasn't changed a great deal, other people, perhaps who are a little bit more removed from him, perceive him as being more capable.

The cochlear implant cannot be expected to change the nature of an implantee's professional qualifications. However, as noted in previous chapters, a properly implemented rehabilitation programme should result in an enhancement of a recipient's employment status, if this is sought.

Concluding remarks

Deafened people presenting at a cochlear implant clinic are seeking much more than a piece of technology to aid deafness. Rather, they are seeking to re-establish themselves in the hearing world and to get on with their lives, however they envisage that outcome to be. Central to the rehabilitative process is the need for the implant clinic to be aware of, and to address, these issues of adjustment to disability and deafness. In the scheme of a client's rehabilitation programme, psychosocial inputs will take up relatively little time and comparatively few resources. They will, however, greatly enhance the ease with which a client moves though the rehabilitation process, enabling them, as it does, to get life back on track. I trust that the ideas and strategies detailed in this book, and in the workshop material contained in the following chapter, will be of some assistance to you in this important work.

Part III
Psychosocial Rehabilitation Programme

CHAPTER 10

A communication skills programme for people with acquired hearing loss

This programme has been adapted from Hearing and Listening Skills Programme, Acoustics Group, University of Montreal. Additional materials have been developed in conjunction with Emma Rushbrooke and Karen Pedley from Queensland Cochlear Implant Clinic, Brisbane and others have been adapted from Christopher Lind's Hear Service Programme, Melbourne. Drawings include Harriet Kaplan's restaurant exercises and my impression of Getty and Hetu's Barbecue exercise that was put into graphic form by Janette Brazel.

Introduction

This chapter outlines a communication skills programme for working with people with an acquired hearing loss. The exercises were developed from the foundational work of Raymond Hetu and Louise Getty at the University of Montreal in Canada. Additional exercises have been adapted from a wide variety of sources and are acknowledged accordingly throughout. The preceding chapters of this text provide the theoretical background for the exercises described here. If you have not read the main text, please go and read it now. You will not be able to implement the exercises successfully without thoroughly understanding this background material.

There is a host of material in this chapter – more than you will be able to get through in any one intervention. The purpose of providing you with extra material is to enable you to move with the clients as you seek to address issues that are of most concern to them. So as each group works

Note: The material in this Chapter may be copied for teaching purposes.

its way through the exercises you will find that you will use some and skip over others. This is fine. Indeed, feel free to move exercises around to suit the needs of your group. However, while doing so keep in mind the pedagogy that underpins the programme:

- problem identification;
- problem exploration;
- problem resolution.

The programme seeks, in a gentle way, to enable clients to recognize the impact of deafness in their lives and on their identity, to begin to appreciate how they may have internalized negative ideas about deafness, and to realize how these ideas hold them back from living a full life. A renewed self-confidence is developed in a threefold process. Individuals (1) become aware of the impact of deafness in their lives, (2) while developing new attitudes towards themselves and others and (3) while developing a new communicative skills set that enables them to begin living their life in a new and proud fashion. It is important therefore, that the initial exercises be taken slowly, giving people time to settle into the experience, to settle any fears they may have about the group process, and to become more comfortable about talking to people in a group setting. Ice breakers are obviously important then so please do not skip over them.

The exercises are intended to be used in a group setting. This means that you will have 6–8 people with hearing loss in the group plus partners. A minimum of three partners is essential if partners are to participate successfully. As many of the exercises pivot on the materials provided by group members, these numbers need to be present in order for the process to work.

To aid you in running the workshops, each exercise has an identified objective, suggested materials and strategies and a suggested time period for the exercise. Some key questions and statements have been **bolded** so that you can refer to them with greater ease. Some exercises, like relaxation training, have quite well-defined time lines. However, TIME is a suggested period for planning purpose. Depending on the group and the level of discussion that emerges, the time will vary greatly. My experience shows that participants enjoy the workshop, it becomes a life-changing experience. I have really enjoyed running the programme – I trust that you will too.

Preparing to run a group: some things to think about

10.1 Preparation

10.1.1 Equipment

You will need the following materials:

(a)	Printed handouts as per each exercise	Yes / No
(b)	Laminated butcher paper prepared with headings for each exercise	Yes / No
(c)	Poster of the ear	Yes / No
(d)	Poster of hair cells (for people with less severe losses)	Yes / No
(e)	Whiteboard	Yes / No
(f)	Whiteboard markers	Yes / No
(g)	Sticky/masking tape/magnets	Yes / No
(h)	TV and video	Yes / No
(i)	Spare sheets of flipchart paper	Yes / No
(j)	Markers	Yes / No
(k)	Overhead projector and pens	Yes / No
(l)	FM or infra-red system	Yes / No
(m)	Assistive devices	Yes / No
(n)	Attachments for cochlear implants/hearing aids	Yes / No
(o)	Hearing help kits[1]	Yes / No
(p)	Tea/coffee/urn/milk,sugar,cups	Yes / No
(q)	Healthy snacks	Yes / No
(r)	Herbal teas/juice/ lots of water	Yes / No
(s)	Name tags	Yes / No

[1]In Australia these kits are referred to as Access 2000 kits and contain a video on accessing various services when you have a hearing loss plus Hearing Help Cards, badges and stickers that depict the WHO blue deafness symbol.

NB: If providing refreshments or lunch, please ensure that healthy alternatives are available. Some of your clients will have diabetes or other health concerns requiring low fat foods.

(Photocopy this page and use is as a check list when preparing facilities and materials for the programme.)

10.2 Setting up

10.2.1 Organizing the room and the surrounding environment

The room should be arranged to facilitate good communication between all group members and the group leaders. Tables and chairs which are set up in a rectangle or square seem to work well. Long narrow rectangles do not seem to work well. It is important therefore, to ensure that the room you pick is large enough in terms of the width as well as depth, i.e. it provides an opportunity for everyone to see each other and that there is space left to walk around the tables and chairs with ease.

Traditionally, people like to set up group meetings in a semi-circular fashion, as this is supposed to promote interaction. My experience is that the group process can be quite confronting from the client's perspective. This is often the first time people have spoken publicly about their hearing difficulties. With these factors in mind, I have found that the tables give people an experience of *space* or safety that aids the group work process. In addition, the tables give people somewhere to put their drinks, their programme handouts and their assistive listening devices. You may be surprised by the amount of water participants consume in any workshop.

It is important that glare is removed from the room, especially in the late afternoons, so curtains may be important. Adequate heating and cooling are also important factors to be considered – participants need to be comfortable.

10.2.2 Before the session

If using an infra-red system or a hearing loop, this should be set up before the group arrives, as would be the refreshments. At the front of the room have the whiteboard, an overhead projector and screen (if using overheads), prepared posters, butcher paper, spare paper, sticking tape and pens ready. The whiteboard or flip chart (a good supply) should be placed at the front of the room but off centre, so that those relying on having things written down can see what is being said. Take care to ensure that light reflecting on the board does not make the board unreadable.

10.3 Suggested overview of workshop sessions

The programme ideally is operated as four 2-hour workshops, plus a brief follow-up workshop 3 months later.

Session 1

1. Introduction: 'What's the worst thing about living with a hearing loss?'
2. The audiogram (for groups with people with less severe hearing loss)
3. Going to a barbecue or birthday party
4. Recognizing the effects of deafness on the body
5. Relaxation exercise I
6. Homework activity (for part-time group) – talking about your deafness

Session 2

7. Review of homework exercise
8. Managing difficult listening situations – going to a restaurant
9. Being assertive: learning to make requests in keeping with one's hearing loss
10. Sorting out roles
11. Role changes

Session 3

12. Identity awareness exercise
13. Assistive listening devices
14. Marion's dinner party
15. Relaxation exercise

Session 4

16. Managing hearing loss in day-to-day interactions
17. More assertiveness training
18. Access 2000 video
19. More strategies for communicating in difficult situations
20. Taking responsibility for my communication needs
21. Managing at work
22. Relaxation exercise
23. Finishing up

Appendices

1. Follow-up letter for writing to participants after the programme
2. Handouts for each session

The workshop

Provide participants with a timetable outlining the sessions for your programme.

Equipment

Distribute assistive listening devices (e.g. FMs). Link up implant/hearing aid users to the loop.

Introductory statements and activities

- Explain the rules for communicating in today's group (see handout below).
- Give the basic outline of the sessions to participants.
- Explain the timetable for the session (including breaks, time for lunch, finish and so on. Highlight healthy alternatives).
- Give information on cost of lunch if appropriate.
- Locate the toilets and safety exists as appropriate.

Handouts

Each participant is given a folder. The folder is to be used to store handouts as the workshop progresses. As a rule, I do not give participants all the handouts at once. This is for several reasons. First, they may get lost (or left at home for the part-time programme). Second, some participants will expect you to follow the programme in the order in which the sheets are printed. Third, people tend to get confused when trying to turn to a particular handout. Finally, you won't be certain which activities you will ultimately use until the group is running.

- Give each couple a file for the session. The file will contain the first handout (Figure 10.1) Explain that during the session they will be given handouts to place in the folder and that if they wish they can follow the programme using the notes provided.
- Emphasize that after the session, the file will help them as a reference when needed.
- Outline the day's programme.

Suggestions to improve communication

It is important to agree on some guidelines to help our communication – the better we communicate, the more effective the whole group process will be and the more we will gain from the whole experience. Below are some suggestions which will be explained in a little more detail. If anyone has anything to add, please do so.

1. **Right to Pass** – while we would encourage you to participate and we value your contribution, it is important that you have the right to choose to participate or to pass. Passing means that you do not have to answer a question if you do not want to.
2. **Mutual Respect** – while you may not always agree with others' views/opinions, it is important to acknowledge them. When giving any feedback, try and give it descriptively rather than judgementally.
3. **One at a Time** – not talking over one another ➠ turn-taking.
   We have a range of hearing abilities in our group; that is, some people hear better than others, so therefore it is very important that only one person speaks at a time.
4. **Confidentiality** – while you can discuss what you've gained and learned from the workshop outside the group, it is important not to refer to people specifically by name. This is important so that people feel safe in expressing ideas and feelings.
5. **I Statements** – speaking for yourself ➠ owning feelings and ideas
6. **Finishing up** – sometimes the group may go off on tangents and we need to agree on a signal we can use which signifies that we need to wind things up. If this sign is made to you then it is time to finish up what you are saying so that we can move on.

Figure 10.1: Rules for the workshop.

Session 1

1. What's the worst thing about having a hearing loss and/or living with a cochlear implant?

OBJECTIVE

The activity which follows is aimed at making the participants aware of the difficulties caused by deafness. At the same time, the session helps to identify the nature and range of concerns to be addressed during the workshop.

THEME: Problem identification.

MATERIALS REQUIRED: Tables and chairs set up in a rectangular fashion. Butcher paper and markers. Masking tape or other sticking material or whiteboard.

TIME: Up to 1 hour.

- Cocktail effect - can't distinguish sounds
- Like words tend to sound the same
- It's just harder to hear now
- Some loud sounds hurt my hearing
- Ringing or buzzing sounds in the ear

Figure 10.2: Key difficulties.

- Can't hear TV/Radio
- Can't hear on the phone
- Can't hear in group settings
- Can't manage difficult situations
- Loss of confidence
- Tinnitus

Figure 10.3: Common problems with hearing loss.

Process

- The facilitator asks each member of the group, starting with the Deafened people, to tell the group what they find most difficult about their deafness. The co-leader writes people's replies on the appropriate space on the poster. If the replies are incomplete, reform the question to better define their difficulties. For the partners, do the same process as for the Deafened people, but this time whilst asking each what they find most difficult about the deafness of their partner, also ask them how they cope with the problem. Support the partners as they express their own difficulties in such a way that they feel that their problems are legitimate.
- Summarize and compare the comments given by participants and partners.
- Without entering into drawn out discussions, show that a real problem exists and that often deaf people tend not to talk about their difficulties. Provide participants with copies of the handouts for this exercise, as a summary of the issues covered today.

Key things to think about while running this session

What issues are raised by particular clients; their comfort levels, apparent barriers or concerns.

State (at the end of this exercise): **The programme is going to:**
- help them better understand the problems they face;
- identify strategies for dealing with these difficulties.

2. The audiogram

Objective

For groups of people with less severe hearing loss, it is often useful to take people through the audiogram. However, in doing so, make sure that the presentation is kept clear and simple. Basically people want to know:

- what the lines on the graph mean;
- how these lines relate to what they can and can't hear.

MATERIALS REQUIRED: A copy of each person's audiogram and an overhead or poster of the audiogram so that each person's audiogram can be drawn up (if they are happy for you to do so).

TIME: Up to 45 minutes.

Process

Place the drawing/overhead of the audiogram up for everyone to see. Then invite a group member to explain what an audiogram means. By having the participants explain as much as they can, it prevents the group leader from going off into a boring lecture on audiograms (we just cannot help ourselves sometimes!). Then invite each person in turn to have their audiogram drawn up. Then ask them (not you) to explain the result as best they can. Fill in the bits they miss and ask them one or two key questions about their listening experience based on their hearing loss (e.g. trouble hearing soft sounds; problems hearing in groups or in background noise). Ask the partners if what they are learning makes sense to them, given their experience of living with the person with this degree of hearing loss.

Have a short break and then introduce the next session.

3. Going to a barbecue or birthday party: recognizing the social impact of hearing loss

Objective

This activity is aimed at provoking a discussion on:

- the social realities of hearing loss;
- the difficulty of making requests because of deafness;
- the social impact of deafness on our partner.

TIME: 45 minutes to 1 hour.

State: **We are now going to do an exercise where we look at a common problem of living with a hearing loss – managing a difficult social situation.**

MATERIALS AND DIRECTIONS: For this activity, the participants are split into two groups, one for people with hearing loss and one for partners. For the people with hearing loss: provide them with a copy of the handout of this exercise 'The Barbecue Birthday Party – People with hearing loss'. Provide the partners with a copy of the handout for exercise 'A Barbecue Birthday Party – partners'. Take your respective group through the scenario described in the handout. Then, using the prompts written below, pose the questions to the group and write down the answers on a piece of paper. Again, make sure everyone participates.

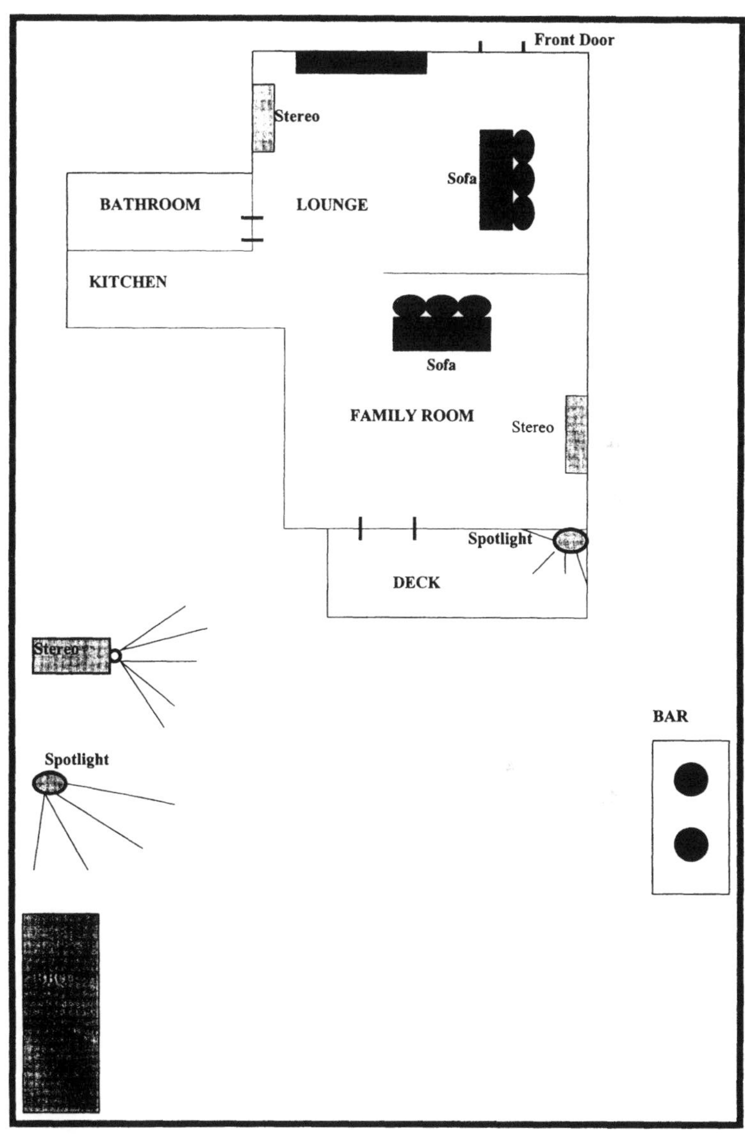

Figure 10.4: Layout of the barbecue party.

- Ann, your sister-in-law, has organized a big barbecue party for your brother's birthday. She has invited you, your partner and also some friends. When you arrive at their home you realize that there are about twenty people present and you do not know many of them. To create a real party atmosphere, for the evening, Ann has installed big outdoor candles all around the backyard and some loud speakers so that people can dance to the music. The food is excellent and the beer very good, people seem to be really enjoying themselves. It is becoming a little loud, it seems that everyone is talking at the same time and because a few people drink a little too much, their speech is more slurred. On top of that, in all the commotion you seem to have lost your partner. You realize that alone it is difficult to follow a conversation, you really did not understand the last joke someone just told. It looked very funny because everybody was laughing.

Figure 10.5: Barbecue birthday party handout for people with hearing loss.

- Ann, your sister-in-law, has organized a big barbecue party for your brother's birthday. She has invited you, your partner and also some friends. When you arrive at their home you realize that there are about twenty people present and you do not know many of them. To create a real party atmosphere, for the evening, Ann has installed big outdoor candles all around the backyard and some loud speakers so that people can dance to the music. The food is excellent and the beer very good, people seem to be really enjoying themselves. It is becoming a little loud, it seems that everyone is talking at the same time and because a few people drink a little too much, their speech is more slurred. You have found yourself chatting to a group away from your partner. You look over and realize that alone your partner is finding it difficult to follow the conversation; your partner clearly missed a joke that was just told. It looked very funny because everybody was laughing.

Figure 10.6: Barbecue birthday party handout for partners.

- Maintain visual contact
- Hold an upright posture
- Begin your sentences with 'I'
- Use short sentences and only say important things
- Try to remain relaxed

Figure 10.7: Strategies which help when talking to people.

- Eliminate the problem
- Assert your needs
- Negotiate a better communication environment
- Reduce noise/improve lighting , etc.
- Situate yourself away from the noise
- Put up with the problem
- Leave early/go home/stay home

Figure 10.8: Strategies for dealing with difficult situations.

- Feeling guilty/frustrated
- Conflict management due to hearing loss
- Having to repeat
- Feeling 'yelled' at
- Noise from TV, etc.

Figure 10.9: Common problems reported by partners.

QUESTIONS FOR GROUP DISCUSSIONS

Ask the people with hearing loss:

(a) which situations they find difficult;
(b) what they would do in each situation;
(c) if they did nothing, why was this so?

In the second group, partners are asked:

(a) in which situations they believe their partners would have difficulties;
(b) what they would do and what they think their partners would do;
(c) why, according to them, they (*people with hearing loss*) would not do anything.

When the discussion has been completed, return to the main group.
Once the exercise has been completed by both groups, bring the two groups back together and explain that we are going to go through everyone's responses together.

First, write on the flipchart the people with hearing loss replies:

- the situations they find difficult;
- what they would do in each situation;
- if they did nothing, why was this so?

Then write down the partners' responses:

- the situation where they believe their partners would have difficulties;
- what they would do and what they think their partners would do;
- why, according to them, they (people with hearing loss) would not do anything.

Ask participants what they think of the results – especially of the partners' responses differing from the people with hearing loss. The most important aspect of the activity depends on the discussion that is going to follow. Encourage people to discuss the difficulties hearing-impaired/deaf people experience and, where appropriate, encourage individuals to admit their difficulties.

Pose the following questions:

- Do they talk openly of these difficulties? If yes, to whom?
- Can one manage without talking about these problems? What would be the consequences of talking about them?
- What would people say about them if they state positively that their deafness is a problem?

Take up the key elements of the discussion and emphasize the positive aspects of informing others (such as family, work, public services/shops, etc.) of their hearing difficulties.

Summary: six steps to managing difficult communication settings

State: **Now that we have covered all the issues concerning managing hearing loss in a difficult setting like a party, let's see if we can identify some ways of overcoming these problems.**
Thinking about the barbecue setting, what could be done so that there were no hearing problems?

Seek out responses from the group and write them up on the board. Now workshop the group with a view to identifying a hierarchy of strategies for preventing and/or managing communication problems. This hierarchy is as follows:

- Eliminate the problem.
- Assert your needs.
- Negotiate a better communication environment (reduce noise/improve lighting, etc.).
- Situate yourself away from the noise.
- Put up with it.
- Go home/stay home.

Emphasize *that the subject 'how to make a request more easily' will be taken up later in the course of the session.*

Recognize *that making requests is difficult and may often be stressful. It is therefore important to recognize the impact that communication may have on the body and our health in general.*

4 Recognizing the impact of deafness on the body: stress

Objective

To enable participants to recognize the impact of hearing-related stress in their lives and begin to enable them to do something (additional) about it.

Process

Discussion and information sharing.

TIME: 15–20 minutes.

State: **Managing stressful and difficult situations could be described as constantly managing uncertainty.** In order to manage difficult situations we need to recognize what is going on at five levels. These are:

(i) within the physical environment;
(ii) at the level of the interpersonal and behavioural – what's happening here?
(iii) how's this occurring?
(iv) who's involved?
(v) what does it feel like?

Refocus for a moment on the barbecue exercise and answer the following questions:

(a) What was it about the barbecue *setting* that makes it difficult for deaf people to communicate?
(b) What was it about people's ***behaviour*** during the barbecue that made it difficult for deaf people to communicate?
(c) Remember what you said you'd do at the barbecue – could the way you communicate add to the problem? (Cite some examples if people are reluctant to speak up.) Could the way others tried to communicate also add to the problem?
(d) Who are the stakeholders in this communication setting? What does deafness mean to them?
(e) How do you feel when you're in a situation like that? How do you think the other people felt when they were talking to you?

Work through people's responses to these questions and then ask the group to answer the following question, but before doing so, encourage them to reflect on the question for a moment:

When you're in a social situation, what do you want to get out of it?*

Elicit comments and then summarize them as goals centred on 'I' statements like:

(a) I feel comfortable when I'm speaking with others.
(b) I enjoy chatting with other people.
(c) I like to get together with people socially.

Now ask participants to **think about the goal underlying their statement – what is their intended outcome from this process?** Examples might be:

(a) I feel a part of what's going on.
(b) I enjoy myself.
(c) I feel happy.

Now ask participants to take this process yet another step further and think again about the goal underlying their statement – what is their **intended outcome** from this process? Examples might be:

(a) I feel I belong – I am one with people.
(b) I know I'm OK.
(c) I am content with myself.

Close this session by noting that often the feelings of ill ease we have are merely the reverse side of a positive goal that we might have. It's important to take a moment to think about what it is we're trying to achieve, perhaps at a deeper level than one first might realize.

Managing stress

AIM

To enable participants to more effectively manage experiences of stress.

MATERIALS: Set of handouts for this exercise on colour-coded paper (see also instructions below). Create handouts for immediate symptoms in colour groups to match long-term conditions of unmanaged stress. For example getting angry and high blood pressure would be colour matched with vascular problems, gas and wind with digestive problems and so on.

---

*Note: this exercise is based on a neurolinguistic counselling strategy and draws on the 10 steps to core transformation documented by Andreas and Andreas (1994).

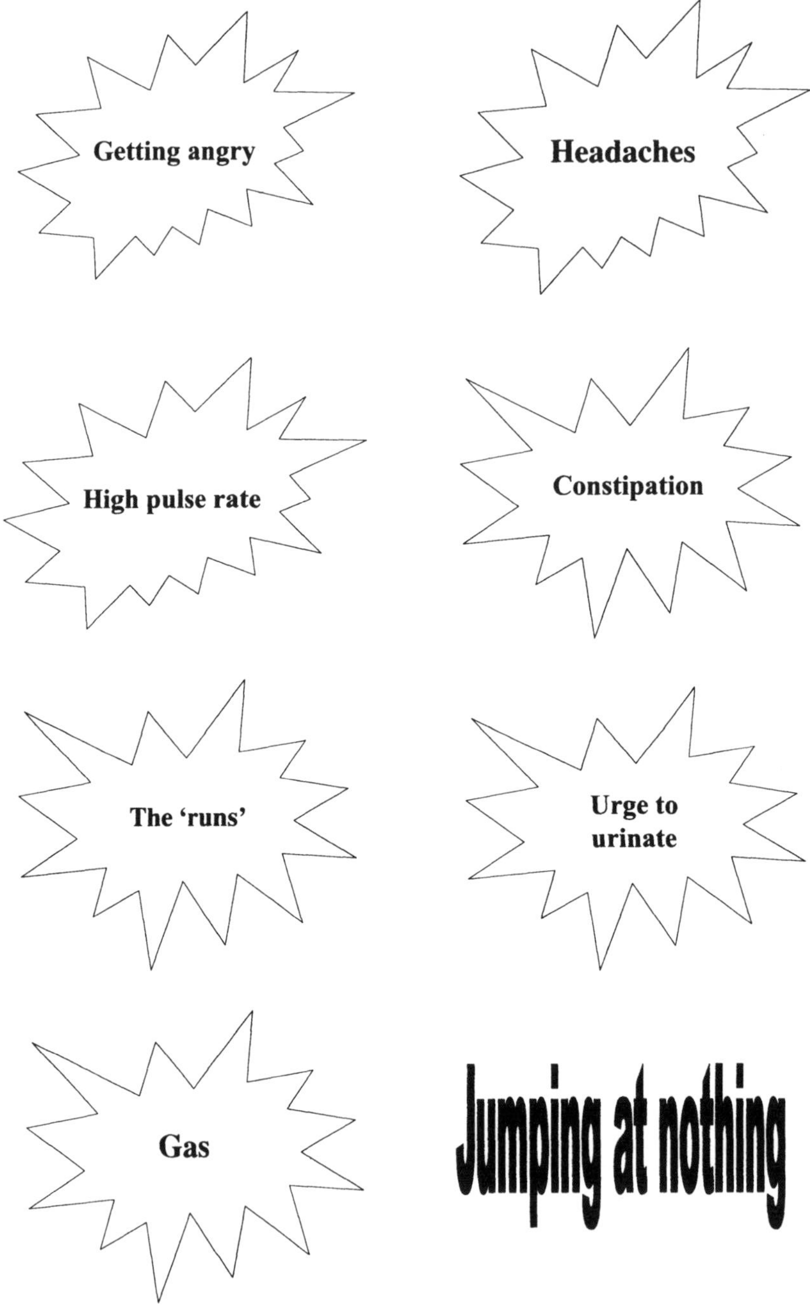

Suggested layouts for stress exercise.

Worrying

Nervy and snappy

Constantly
on edge

aches

muscle tension

stiffness

High blood pressure

Depression
less agreeable life

Suggested handouts for stress exercise.

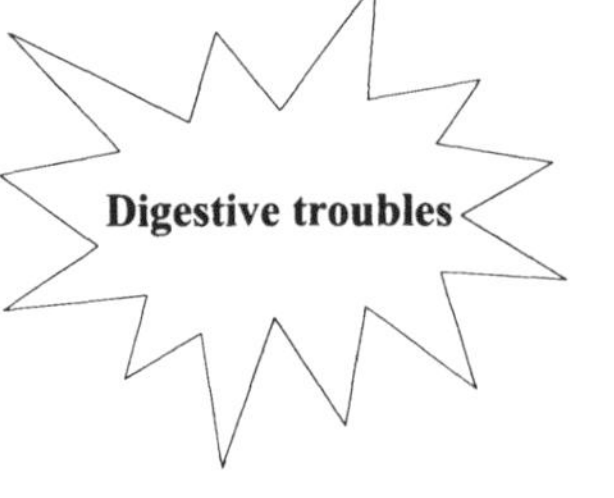

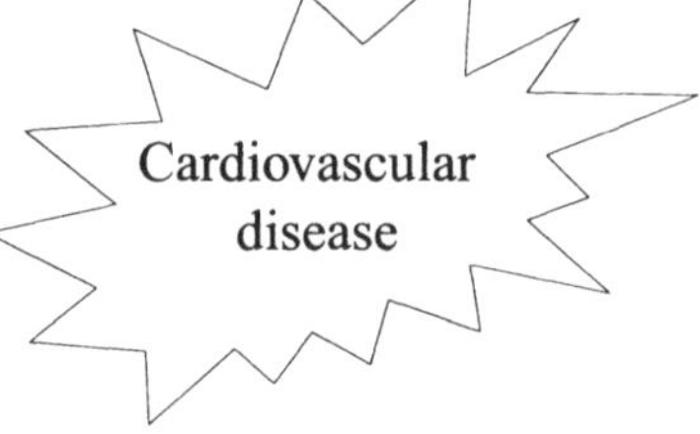

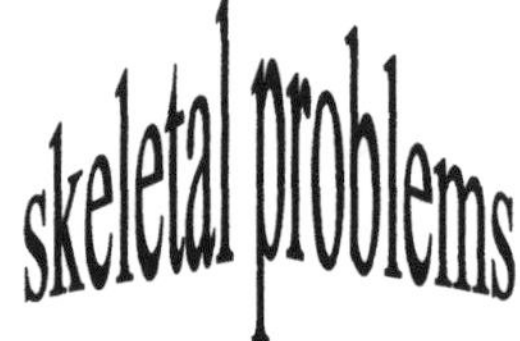

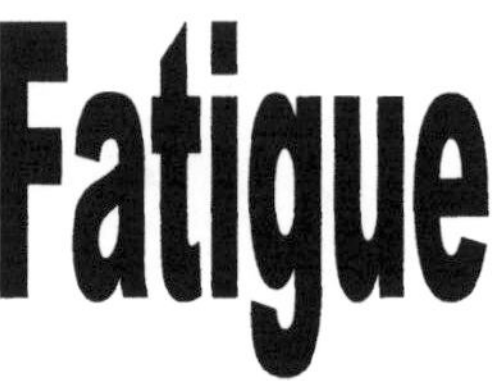

Suggested handouts for stress exercise.

Objective

At the end of this session participants will be able to:

(a) identify physical indicators of stress;
(b) relate indicators of stress to longer-term health problems;
(c) develop an understanding of the relationship between emotion and stress;
(d) identify strategies for learning to relax;
(e) practise a relaxation exercise.

State: **So far we have seen that hearing loss creates difficulties for us in our day-to-day lives. One of these difficulties is feeling stressed, tense or just physically uncomfortable.**

- Ask each participant in turn – '**how would you know if you were feeling stressed?**' Note the list of symptoms highlighted (e.g. headaches, neck pain, etc.).
- Distribute around the room, cards listing various types of stress symptoms (see left-hand column of Table 10.1). Ask participants to identify the symptoms they experience most often.

Table 10.1: Signs and symptoms of stress - key concepts

Immediate Signs	**Long-term effects**
feeling really agitated more nervous jumping at nothing get angry more quickly become less tolerant	unstable depressive less agreeable life
high pulse rate high blood pressure	cardiac problems vascular problems (hypertension)
greater muscular tension	fatigue various ills (eg back)
lessening of digestive functions	digestive troubles (e.g. ulcers)

- Once this is done, the group leader gathers up the cards and goes through each one, encouraging participants to identify which symptom, if any, is theirs. As they do so, they are given the card they identify with. If more than one person identifies with the symptom, encourage them to sit together.
- Once all the cards are given out, the leader goes through the longer-term consequences of the symptoms which have been written on pieces of cardboard of the same colour as the symptoms. The use of colour coding assists participants to make the connection between long-term and short-term experiences of stress. By grouping people with similar difficulties together, the experience of stress is demystified as stress is seen as something common to group members.
- Note that the body holds stress and that it needs to be released on a regular basis. Holding on to emotion may result in health problems in the longer term. You might also like to describe unresolved stress as slowly building up the body's alert system. As stress is experienced over time the body moves from being generally in a relaxed state to being permanently a little on edge to being permanently quite a lot on edge and so on. Note also that by regularly relaxing the body we are able to reduce this state of alert back to one that is resting, stable and calm.
- Ask participants to identify the ways symptoms of stress show up in our daily lives. Note that each experience of stress may be different for each person (some examples are listed below).

Stress indicators

Table 10.2: Some indicators of feeling stressed

breathing changes (shorter)	sweating
sweating hands	dizzy
dry throat	stomach ache
head aches	urge to urinate
moving about quickly	avoiding things
difficulty sleeping	bad digestion
pupils dilate	

Also, ask participants if they noticed that particular foods or drinks made them feel stressed.

Note that the following substances contribute to stress and fatigue:

- caffeine
- alcohol
- cane sugar
- high fat foods
- no/little exercise
- lack of sleep
- over-active stimuli (e.g. TV that winds you up before bedtime; watching suspense movies for relaxation).

Note: Part of getting rid of stress out of your life is to detoxify the body, but this is best done under the guidance of a health professional. Some natural therapists specialize in this type of work (e.g. naturopath, acupuncturist, herbalist, some chiropractors). However, it can be dangerous to simply change one's eating, drinking habits, or to take up a new exercise regime without the support and supervision of such a person.

Ask participants, in turn, what do you do to relax?
Create a list of activities. They might include:

- various types of exercise
- relaxation exercises
- walking
- diet
- yoga
- tai chi
- meditation
- prayer

- crafts
- hobbies
- sport (active and passive)
- junk movies/novels
- gardening
- herbs
- aromatherapy
- oil baths/showers
- massage.

Emphasize that relaxation can be active or passive and does not necessarily involve spending money, or a lot of it. A relaxing bath with lavender oil might cost very little – a walk costs nothing at all.

5. Relaxation exercise 1

Observe: **Getting people to accommodate your deafness is difficult. It is therefore important to recognize the impact that communication may have on the body and health in general. In this exercise I want you to think about being out of balance, as though the scales were tipped to one extreme or the other. Stress has this effect in our lives of tipping our bodies and/or our minds out of balance. It is important, therefore, to take steps that bring your life back into balance. A way of overcoming this feeling of being out of balance is by learning how to relax on a regular basis.**

A relaxation exercise, such as slow breathing or the Jacobsen method (progressive muscle relaxation) is then undertaken.

Then take a break or end the session.

Recall

Briefly go over what has been covered so far:

- what hearing loss is;
- problems arising from a hearing loss;
- ways of reducing the effects of stress on the body.

Conclusion

If the session is being run on a weekly basis – give participants the homework exercise below.

6. Homework

Aim

The purpose of this exercise is to encourage participants to discuss their hearing loss with people outside the group process.

MATERIALS: Handout for homework exercise (see Figure 10.10).

PEOPLE WITH HEARING LOSS: Encourage the people with hearing loss to complete the homework exercise listed below. It is to be presented at the next meeting (their partners may help them). They must:

1. choose a close acquaintance (child, parent, friend, neighbour or other) and tell them that they are attending a readjustment meeting for their hearing problem;
2. try to explain to this person how hearing loss effects their communication and tell the person what makes communication easier for them.

PARTNERS: The homework for the partners of the hearing-impaired person is as follows:

The partner is to try to be aware of the times he or she 'rescues' the people with hearing loss in difficult communication situations. If possible, discuss these situations with your partner. Was he or she aware of what happened? How did he or she react when you pointed out to him or her that you 'helped' out? Was there another way the situation could have been managed?

- 1. Choose a person from around you such as a child, parent, neighbour, friend or other person and tell them that you are attending a readjustment meeting for your hearing problem
- 2. Try to explain to this person something of what you learnt about the effects of hearing loss in the lives of deafened people.
- To help you with the explanations, you can use the handouts from the programme.

Figure 10.10: Handout for homework exercise.

Session 2

7. Review of homework exercise

RECALL 1: Go over what participants had to do for homework and pose the following questions, moving around the group to see how everyone fared:

- What did they do?
- How did it go?
- Difficulties encountered?
- Equipment used?
- Questions posed by the partner?
- The reaction of the partner?
- What did the partner get out of it?

Congratulate them on the effort they put into the activity. Acknowledge that the exercise was challenging.

RECALL 2: Briefly go over what has been covered during the last session:
- what hearing loss is;
- the problems arising from a hearing loss;
- the ways of reducing the effects of stress on the body.

8. Managing difficult listening situations: going to a restaurant

Introduce what will be coming in this session:
- identifying and managing communication in difficult settings;
- more on relaxation.

Objective

To enable people to identify problematic communication settings and to practise strategies for managing these.

MATERIALS: Hand out copies of the restaurant exercise (Figure 10.11) to participants.

TIME: 45 minutes.

Process

Observe: **Managing hearing difficulties in social settings can be difficult. In today's exercise, we are going to look at issues of communicating in one social setting – a restaurant.**

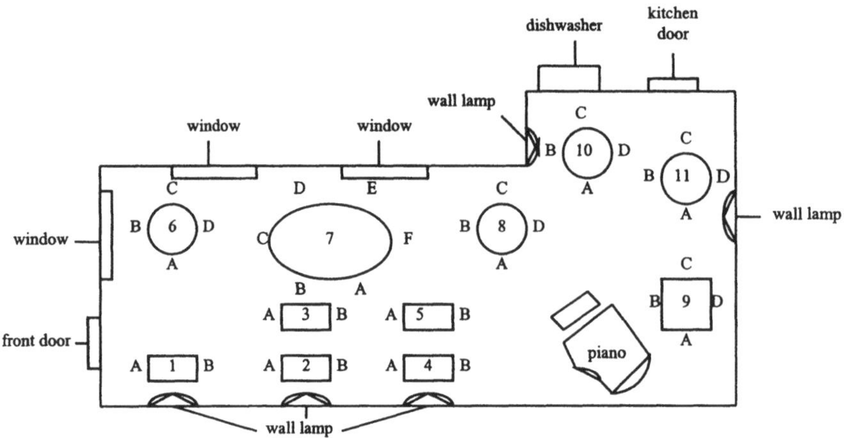

Source: adapted from Kaplan, Bally and Garrestson (1985).

Figure 10.11: Hearing tactics: a restaurant.

- Lead participants through the exercise in the usual manner, having respondent's identify the communication hazards, the better tables to sit at and so on. Then rework the dynamics of the exercise as described in Chapter 5.
- Have participants identify where they would like to sit and why.
- Begin to role-play the situation, assuming that you are the Maître d'Hotel.
- Place participants at tables of your choosing.
- Ask them – would they be happy there at this table? Would they sit there if directed to do so? How would they feel about having to sit there? What would happen to their body, their stress responses? What could they do to overcome these difficulties?
- Work the group to highlight the various communication barriers and problems present in the restaurant and then move on to practise 'I' statements; assertively expressing their needs.
- Talk with people about their statements when such statements are passive or aggressive. Allow the group to feel the difficulty of resolving this situation. However, if they look as though they are getting really stuck, remind them of the hierarchy and begin to resolve the situation this way.
- For example, ask them what could be done to ensure that you have a good time when you go out to dinner (e.g. plan ahead, find a good, quiet restaurant, etc.)?

- *Note*: at this time participants will say things such as: I will sit there and put up with it, I would say nothing and so on. It is important at this time to emphasize the point that they would be paying money here, to have a bad time, to be stressed, or marginalized. Ask people if this is really what they want. Clearly it is not.
- Then role-play solutions with respondents. By role-playing I do not mean getting up and walking about the room (though this is fine if people are comfortable to do so), simply having people making requests, in keeping with their hearing loss is all that is required. This means having people say: 'I do not like this table, I am hearing-impaired/deaf and I will not be able to hear well at this table. I would like such and such a table' (or a similar statement). However, most people, when beginning 'I' statements will skirt around this issue by saying things such as – I'm a bit deaf. A bit deaf! This is poor communication and gives the communication partner the entirely wrong message.
- Clarify these issues with participants and work with them as they make correct and accurate statements abut their hearing needs. Encourage other deafened participants to suggest solutions. Create dilemmas for individuals to solve.
- For example, a participant might appropriately request Table Six. Tell them that Table Six is taken – make them work for what they want – for if they will not make appropriate requests in the safety of the group – they certainly will not do so outside in the real world. Then, move on to identifying strategic ways of avoiding problems (e.g. booking ahead, eating at restaurants that offer easy access to communication).

When you have finished the exercise, affirm and congratulate participants for their efforts, recognizing how difficult it may be for them, while reinforcing how many of these difficulties can be minimized or eliminated.

Have a break.

9. Being assertive: learning to make requests in keeping with one's hearing loss

Objective

This activity is aimed at recognizing and experimenting with ways which enable participants to make requests in keeping with their hearing loss by practising assertiveness.

MATERIALS: Provide participants with a copy of the handout for this exercise: Responding to challenging situations 1 (the doctor's waiting room) (Figure 10.12).

- You have been sitting in your doctor's waiting room for nearly an hour past your appointment time. People who have arrived after you have been seen by your doctor. The receptionist at the desk seems to be unaware of your lengthy wait. You decide to:
- Passive____
- ____
- Aggressive:____
- ____
- Assertive:____
- ____

Source: adapted from an original design by Christopher Lind, Victorian Hearing Service – used with permission.

Figure 10.12: Responding to challenging situations 1 – the doctor's waiting room.

PROCESS

Structured discussions.

TIME: 45 minutes to 1 hour.

EXPLANATION I: Explain that with the solutions that have been covered so far, several require that when making a request, you have to say that you have a hearing problem. Emphasize that the exercises to follow are aimed at improving their ability to make the requests. Note that the group has already successfully completed a number of these tasks.

Underline the fact that it is important to make requests according to your needs.

Observe: **being assertive means expressing clearly what one expects from the other person**.

- Make clear the distinction that asserting oneself is expressing one's needs and not imposing oneself aggressively.
- By questioning, explain what could impede the making of a request (see below).

Ask participants to:

- think about a situation in which they have difficulty asking people to communicate with them;
- observe what it is about the situation that makes them hesitate to make an appropriate request?

The main themes will include:

- because I am too embarrassed;
- because I am afraid of the response from others;
- because I do not know how to make a request.

EXPLANATION II: Explain that making an appropriate request is a whole of body experience. You need to:

- maintain visual contact;
- stand in an upright posture – don't let your feet be too close together;
- begin each sentence with 'I';
- use short sentences;
- be relaxed.

Workshop participants are to try and define the difference between being passive, aggressive and assertive (Robert Bolton's text *People Skills* (Bolton, 1987) provides an excellent background to assertiveness training). Now, having defined these issues, present participants with the scenario of waiting in the doctor's surgery way past your appointment time. How will you manage this situation? What would you do? Allow participants to speak about it briefly. Then move them into role-playing being passive, aggressive and then assertive. Ensure everyone has a chance at being assertive.

10. Sorting out our roles

This exercise is particularly important for helping partners and new implantees talk about their changing roles. However, it will also work well with new hearing aid users who are also beginning to reconnect themselves into communication and who are taking responsibility for their communication needs.

Objective

This activity is aimed at provoking discussion on the role of partners in managing communication breakdown. In particular, the exercise is designed to:

(a) highlight how the Deafened people might rely on their partners for communication;
(b) begin to give both people permission to renegotiate roles now that people have received help for their hearing;
(c) recognize the support the partner has offered in the past while enabling the Deafened person to become more independent.

Process

For this activity, the participants are split into two groups; people with hearing loss and partners.

TIME: 45 minutes.

MATERIALS: Provide participants with a copy of the handout for this exercise and read through the senarios for clients and partners and then work through the questions below in separate groups.

- You and your partner have decided to purchase a holiday. You've been looking at brochures for a while now and have finally decided on a place you would like to go to. You go to visit a travel agent to get more information about your chosen destination and to ask about special offers and prices. As the travel agent begins to answer your questions he is distracted by some other activity in the agency and begins to turn away as he answers you. Consequently, you found it difficult to follow the information you were given.

Figure 10.13: Choosing a holiday – people with hearing loss.

- You and your partner have decided to purchase a holiday. You've been looking at brochures for a while now and have finally decided on a place you would like to go to. You go to visit a travel agent to get more information about your chosen destination and to ask about special offers and prices. As the travel agent begins to answer your questions he is distracted by some other activity in the agency and begins to turn away as he answers you. Consequently, your partner found it difficult to follow the information you were given.

Figure 10.14: Choosing a holiday – partners.

Pose the following questions to the people with hearing loss.

- Have you been in a situation like this before?
- What steps can YOU take so that you could clarify what the sales assistant said to you?
- If your partner intervenes on your behalf, what appropriate ways are there to relay to your partner that you would prefer to try to manage without assistance?

Encourage everyone to participate.

Pose the following questions to the partners' group.

- Have you been in a situation like this before?
- What are the signs that your partner may be expecting you to help out?
- How can you help your partner without reducing their level of responsibility in regards to obtaining the information requested in the first place?

Encourage everyone to participate.

Once the exercise has been completed for both groups, bring the two groups together and explain that we are going to go through everyone's responses as a group on the whiteboard.

Praise the group for their efforts. Summarize the key factors that could potentially impair communication (e.g. noisy shopping centre, assistant turns away). Summarize the behaviours of the hearing-impaired people that suggest that they are withdrawing from the communication (e.g. looking at partner, closed body language like moving closer to you, leaving long pauses, facial expression).

Highlight the strategies suggested by the people with hearing loss for staying in the conversation (e.g. asking for repetition, restating what they thought the travel agent had said, asking for the prices to be written down, maintaining eye contact with the travel agent, not looking to the partner for clarification, not nodding when you are unsure what has been said).

Summarize the strategies suggested by the partners to encourage their hearing-impaired person to take responsibility (e.g. avoid eye contact with the sales assistant, standing back, looking at the hearing-impaired person rather than the travel agent, not asking the travel agent for repetition, asking questions in another way to provide redundancy for partner's benefit).

11. Role changes

Objective

In this exercise participants explore role changes that have occurred as a result of deafness or interventions.

MATERIALS: Large sheets of paper and pens.

Process

Divide into two groups: (1) people with hearing loss; (2) partners.

TIME: 45 minutes.

For people with hearing loss

Ask them to discuss the following points and write answers on a flipchart or big sheets of paper:

- The roles that they gave up as a result of their deafness (e.g. prior to hearing aid/implantation).
- Roles that they have resumed after receiving the implant.
- Those roles that are still carried out by their partner.
- Why are some roles difficult to resume?
- How do they feel about some of the role changes that persist?

For partners

Discuss the following points and write down answers on sheets of paper.

- The roles they took over as their partners lost their hearing, or began to withdraw.
- The roles that they lost because of deafness.
- How they may have encouraged the implantees to resume some of their roles after implantation.
- How did/do they feel about the additional responsibilities?
- Roles that they have lost since their partner got their implant/hearing aid.
- Conflicts that have arisen since help arrived.
- How do they feel about their role in the family now?

Bring the two groups together to discuss all the answers. Highlight the fact that some positive changes occurred after implantation. Note that some roles cannot be resumed. Summarize some of the ways in which implantees have been successfully encouraged to resume former roles. Emphasize the important role that the partners have played, the many changes that they have made following the onset of deafness and following interventions like implantation. Notice how these changes are likely to continue for a while yet.

ASK: Have couples talked about these changes? Perhaps they may, following the group.

Session 3

12. Identity awareness exercise

AIM: The aim of this exercise is to enable participants to identify positive aspects of living with a hearing loss and a cochlear implant/hearing aid.

Note: This exercise is most suitable for a group that is more positively disposed to living with hearing loss. However, it may also be useful for a group that is too focused on the negatives of deafness and that needs to be challenged to move on.

Objective

At the end of this session participants will be able to:

(a) identify positive aspects of having a hearing loss;
(b) discuss these things with other group members;
(c) create an image that symbolizes this experience.

MATERIALS: Old magazines, sheets of paper, lists of feeling words (positive and negative), pens, scissors and sticky tape or glue.

TIME: 1 hour

Process

Break participants into groups of 3–4 people (partners and people with hearing loss separate). For Deafened adults, direct them to create a collage. The theme of this collage is what I like about being deaf. For partners, direct them to create a collage. The theme of this collage is **what I like about living with someone who's deaf/hearing-impaired**. Allow participants 15–20 minutes to create their collages, adjust time frame to suit the needs of the group. When participants are ready (or near enough to being finished) invite them back to the larger group and have them present their work.

Praise the group for their efforts. As people proceed with their presentations, draw attention to key words and phrases used. **Summarize** the themes arising from the posters where they are apparent (e.g. second chance is a common theme). Don't be surprised if there is no apparent or coherent theme across all posters. Rather, highlight the diversity of ideas.

13. Assistive listening devices

Objective

To explore the varied ways in which cochlear implant accessories or assistive listening devices can be used to increase hearing and communication benefits for everyone.

This activity is to be done as a whole group. However, individual follow-up work on specific technologies may be useful too.

Note: Allow for the fact that various participants may bring along new or interesting devices to show the group. It is my experience that certain group members will have enormous expertise in the area of assistive technologies and may have held roles as technology educators in their respective self-help groups. Utilize such group members wherever possible, allowing the group to benefit from their knowledge and experience.

TIME: 45 minutes to an hour.

MATERIALS: A magnetic board with each of the following accessories in turn:

- lapel microphone;
- TV adaptor;
- Walkman/Hi-fi cable.

Magnetized pictures/photographs of communication situations:

- conversing in a car;
- conversing at the bar or a coffee shop;
- conversing across a table in a restaurant;
- meetings;
- hearing the radio in the car;
- listening to CDs;
- listening to a radio talk;
- watching TV;
- family gathering;
- talking to a person sitting next to you in a cinema/theatre;
- answering the telephone;
- computer games;
- CD-Rom encyclopaedia;
- some blank magnetized pictures for people to draw their own.

Discuss which accessories can be used with each situation and vice versa by placing the situation photo by the accessory on the board.

Encourage people to contribute their own experiences, solutions and innovations e.g. shakeawake alarms, visual alert systems, TTYs, fax machine, captioning.

14. Marion's dinner party

Objective

To practise skills for managing difficult listening and social situations.

Process

This exercise is run in a similar fashion to the barbecue exercise. This time, however, participants are expected to show a higher level of problem-solving and to make appropriate 'I' statements in accordance with their needs.

TIME: 45 minutes.

MATERIALS: Provide participants with copies of handouts for this exercise, Figures 10.15–10.17. The handouts are prompt sheets for **Marion's dinner party** and a layout of the dining room.

> Marion, your partner's cousin, likes entertaining a lot. It will soon be her husband's birthday and she wants to make the most of this and organize a big celebratory dinner. And of course she invites you and your partner. You arrive at Marion's, she introduces you to the people you don't know and soon afterwards invites you to go to the dinner. As she has decided to mix everyone up, she assigns a place for you away from your partner. You find youself three places away, between Marion and someone you don't know. Marion wanted to create a good atmosphere, so she has subdued lights and has background music playing on their new compact disc player. To decorate the table she has candles and a large bouquet of flowers, which just happens to be in front of your place. The meal is good, the beer is cold and the wine excellent. Everyone is having a good time, things are warming up and everyone seems to be talking at once. There are some who have had a fair bit to drink and they talk more quickly and less distinctively than at the start of the evening. Marion, who knows you have difficulty hearing tries to say something to you, speaking very slowly and exaggerating her pronunciation; the person next to you looks at her and seems to wonder what is going on. You hasten to change the subject...

Figure 10.15: Marion's dinner party – handout for people with hearing loss.

> Marion, your cousin, likes entertaining a lot. It will soon be her husband's birthday and she wants to make the most of this and organize a big celebratory dinner. And of course she invites you and your partner. You arrive at Marion's, she introduces you to the people you don't know and soon afterwards invites you to go to the dinner. As she had decided to mix everyone up, she assigns a place for you away from your partner. You find yourself three places away, and your partner is between Marion and someone you don't know. Marion wanted to create a good atmosphere, so she has subdued lights and has background music playing on their new compact disc player. To decorate the table she has candles and a large bouquet of flowers, which just happens to be in front of your partner. The meal is good, the beer is cold and the wine excellent. Everyone is having a good time, things are warming up and everyone seems to be talking at once. There are some who have had a fair bit to drink and they talk more quickly and less distinctively than at the start of the evening. Marion, who knows your partner has difficulty hearing, tries to say something to your partner, speaking very slowly and exaggerating her pronunciation; the person next to your partner looks at her and seems to wonder what is going on. Your partner hastens to change the subject...

Figure 10.16: Marion's dinner party – handout for partners.

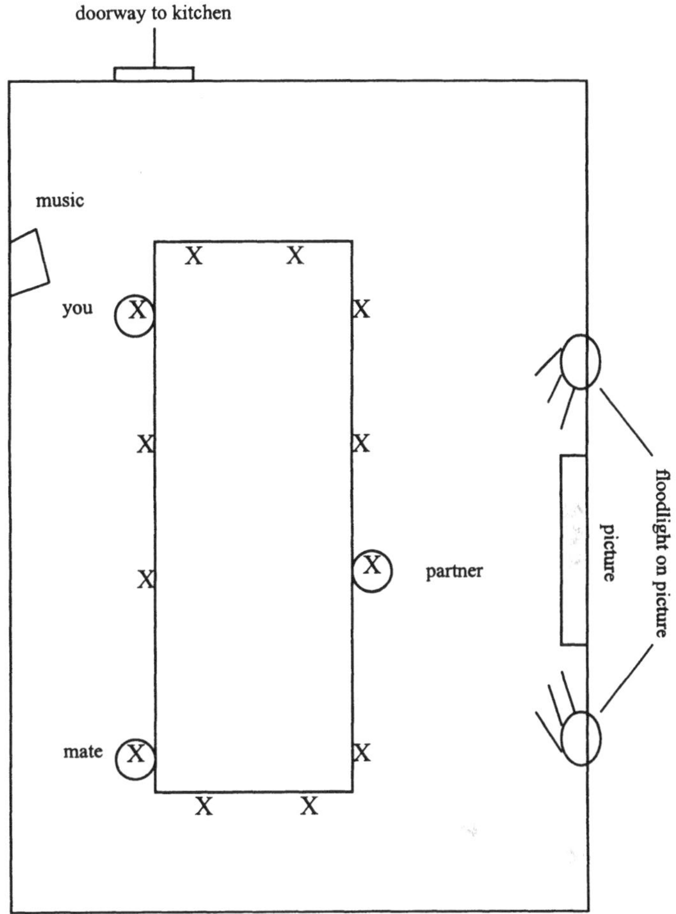

Figure 10.17: Marion's dinner party.

Questions (people with hearing loss)

- What happens to you in these kind of situations?
- What can you do in such situations?
- What don't you do? What are the consequences of doing nothing?

Questions (partners)

- What happens to your partner in situations like this?
- What does he or she usually do in these situations?
- According to you, what could or should he or she do?
- Do you think your partner will do this? If not, why do you think he or she won't do this?

15. Relaxation exercise

Objective

To enhance participants' knowledge of ways to relax

Once again, as the session draws to a close, participants are introduced to a new relaxation exercise. This time – one form of deep breathing.

Process

Take people through a relaxation exercise.

MATERIALS: Provide participants with handout on relaxation, Figure 10.18.

- Focus on point 1" below navel in the middle of your body
- Breathe deeply
- Expand lower abdomen as you breathe in
- Flatten abdomen as you breathe out
- Do for 10–20 minutes

Figure 10.18: Relaxation exercise.

TIME: 20 minutes.

Observe: In sports sciences, trainers refer to the idea of muscle memory. Muscle memory refers to the capacity of a muscle to develop a response set or reflex action to particular stimuli. Strategies for holding or swinging a tennis racquet or managing a bowling ball may be experienced as cumbersome when a person first begins a sport. But as one becomes familiar with the back-hand grip, say in tennis, it becomes progressively easier and eventually quite natural, to hold the racquet in a particular fashion. Relaxing the body follows a similar learning pattern. At first relaxation exercises appear to be cumbersome, odd or awkward, but as the body becomes more familiar with them, it will also respond in a rapid and appropriate fashion.

Today's relaxation exercise appears to be overly simple at first glance. It is simply deep breathing. Even with this initial practice, you should feel some level of deep relaxation after 15–20 minutes of the exercise. With regular practice, however, you will find that you will slip quickly into a relaxed state and that, over time, this level of relaxation will deepen.

Begin the exercise by sitting upright in your chair. Take a moment to think about how you are feeling at present. Notice any points of tension.

Now, about one inch below the navel is a small divot or notch – see if you can find it or as close as you can get. Then, close your eyes and focus on a point inside the body that is level with this spot and in the centre of the body. Commence breathing slowly and deeply, through the nose, focusing your mind on this point. Continue to do so for 20 minutes. You will find that your mind will wander off sometimes, each time this occurs, simply refocus your mind back on the point – known as the Dan Tien or lower energy point – and continue to breath slowly.

When you have finished, take a moment to notice how you're feeling now.

Close.

Session 4

Recall

Briefly go over what has been covered in the programme to date:

- the difficulties of living with a hearing loss;
- ways of facilitating communication.

To come: announce what will be covered in the coming session:

- more ideas on facilitating communication in difficult situations

16. Managing hearing loss in day-to-day interactions

Objective

To practise asserting oneself in difficult listening situations.

MATERIALS: Provide participants with a copy of the handout for this exercise – Responding to challenging situations 2 (making an appointment at the dentist), Figure 10.19.

TIME: 20–30 minutes.

- You have just come out of your appointment with the dentist and you need to make a new time. Your ask the receptionist for a time. She says something to you, but you're not sure what it was she said.
- Passive____________________
- ____________________
- Aggressive:____________________
- ____________________
- Assertive:____________________
- ____________________

Source: adapted from an original design by Christopher Lind, Victorian Hear Service – used with permission.

Figure 10.19: Responding to challenging situations 2 – making an appointment at the dentist.

17. More assertiveness training

Objective

To practise managing communication in difficult settings.

MATERIALS: Responding to challenging situations 3 – at the bank, Figure 10.20.

TIME: 20–30 minutes.

Role-play this scenario with the group, providing each participant with the opportunity to assert themselves and to make 'I' statements. Encourage group members to respond to each person's efforts. Did they find it assertive, passive or aggressive?

- You find yourself waiting in line at a local bank. In this bank the tellers stand behind bullet-proof glass. Each customer window is fitted with a microphone system and some have loops fitted. However, the staff rarely use any of the technology provided. In consequence, it is very difficult to communicate with the bank's staff.
- What 'I' statement could you make here to assert your communication needs with the bank?

Source: adapted from an original design by Christopher Lind, Victorian Hear Service – used with permission.

Figure 10.20: Responding to challenging situations 3 – at the bank.

Acknowledge

- the positive approaches some people take in communicating with people with hearing loss;
- discrimination does exist;
- there are things we can do to make communication flow reasonably easily.

Ask: How did the participants feel when they were practising their assertive statements?

If you haven't already done so – have a break.

Briefly revise the materials covered so far and draw conclusions about the difficulty of talking openly about hearing loss and some advantages of doing it:

- people tend to accommodate you when they understand your needs;
- communication improves;
- you gain satisfaction from interacting with others.

18. Access 2000

Objective

To raise participants' expectations about the quality of service they can expect to receive when dealing with people such as bank officers.

MATERIALS: Access 2000 video, television monitor, video player, assistive devices for TV listening.

TIME: 30 minutes (video: 16 minutes).

Process

Show the Access 2000 video and discuss the ways public service officers are trained to assist communication for people who have a hearing loss.

19. More strategies for communicating in difficult settings

Objective

To enable participants to utilize less direct strategies for managing difficult communication settings

MATERIALS: Hearing Help Cards, deafness stickers and lapel badges from Access 2000 kit.

Hearing Help Kits may be purchased by self-help groups for the hard of hearing.

TIME: 15 minutes.

Process

- *Present* the Hearing Help Cards and *explain that they can be used to give precise information about their hearing loss so that they can use the services best adapted for deaf and hearing-impaired people.*

- *Present* the self-adhesive stickers with the deafness symbol and ***explain that they can be put in appropriate places to ensure a better service***. Example, if in hospital, they can be stuck on your file and daily charts. *Hand out* a Hearing Help Card and stickers to each person.
- Draw a *conclusion* on the numerous aids available to deaf people (training of staff, cards, telephones with couplers, etc) and that if they want an adequate service it is important that they inform the service provider of their hearing problem.
- *Ask* people how they'd *feel* about following the communication strategies outlined in the video. What would they find difficult? In which situations (of the problematic ones they noted in the very first session) could they see themselves following strategies and effectively managing difficult communication settings

20. Taking responsibility for my communication needs

Objective

To enable the Deafened person to take greater responsibility for their communication needs

MATERIALS: Provide participants with copies of the handout for this session (managing communication with your doctor), Figures 10.21–10.22.

TIME: 20–30 minutes.

PROCESS: For this activity, the participants are once again split into two groups, people with hearing loss and partners.

For the people with hearing loss, present the following scenario and then work through the questions below in separate groups.

- You and your partner are attending the doctors to find out the results of some tests you have had and to discuss a management plan for your health. The doctor is running late and appears flustered. You have had to wait a couple of months to see this doctor. The medical condition has been worrying you and you realise this is an important opportunity to sort things out. You are finding it difficult to follow the information you are being given.

Figure 10.21: Taking responsibility – people with hearing loss.

Pose the following questions to the hearing-impaired group:

- What factors here could impair communication?
- What steps can YOU to take so that you can understand the doctor's information?
- If your partner intervenes on your behalf, what appropriate ways are there to relay your partner that you would prefer to try to manage without their assistance?

Encourage everyone to participate.

- You and your partner are attending the doctors to find out the results of some tests your partner has had and to discuss a management plan for your partner's health. The doctor is running late and appears flustered. You have had to wait a couple of months to see this doctor. The medical condition has been worrying your partner and you realise this is an important opportunity to sort things out. Your partner is finding it difficult to follow the information they are being given.

Figure 10.22: Taking responsibility – partners.

Pose the following questions to the partners' group.

- What factors here could impair communication?
- What are the signs that your partner may be expecting you to help out?
- How can you help your partner without reducing their level of responsibility in regards to obtaining the medical information and guidance?

Encourage everyone to participate.

Once the exercise has been completed by both groups, bring the two groups together and explain that we are going to go through responses as a group on the whiteboard.

Praise the group for their efforts. *Summarize* the *key factors* that could potentially impair communication (e.g. busy doctor looking for a quick way out, stress-related importance of issue, unfamiliar medical terms).

Summarize the *behaviours* of the hearing-impaired persons that suggest that they are *withdrawing* from the communication (e.g. looking at partner, closed body language like sitting back, leaving long pauses, facial expression).

Highlight the strategies suggested by the hearing-impaired group for staying in the conversation (e.g. pulling chair closer, asking for repetition, restating what they thought the doctor had said, asking for difficult medical terms to be written down, asking the doctor to draw diagrams, maintaining eye contact with the doctor, not looking to the partner for clarification, not nodding when you are unsure what has been said).

Summarize the *strategies suggested by the partners* to encourage their hearing-impaired person to take responsibility (e.g. avoid eye contact with the doctor, sitting back, looking at the hearing-impaired person, not asking the doctor for repetition, asking questions in another way to provide redundancy for partner's benefit).

21. Managing at work

Objective

To practise managing difficult communication in the workplace.

MATERIALS: Provide participants with a copy of the handout for this exercise (managing at work), Figure 10.23.

- You work in a small office and regularly take material into your supervisor for discussion. The supervisor has a small office and you usually sit opposite her when you go in to see her. Although the supervisor has been trained in communicating with you, she is not very sympathetic to your needs and quickly gets impatient with you. On this occasion, you take an important piece of work into the supervisor that you have been working on for some time. You are keen to impress on the supervisor how well you've done with this project. The supervisor looks at it, starts to write on what you have done and makes comments to you about it. Unfortunately, you missed most of what she said as she was looking down as she spoke, and she had her hand over her head (as if to concentrate). To make matters worse, the photocopy machine, which is just outside the door, was running, making it more difficult for you to hear. The supervisor looks up at you (somewhat sternly) as though she were waiting for you to respond to whatever it was she said.

Figure 10.23: Managing at work.

TIME: 20–30 minutes.

Process

Role-play scenario plus discussion and problem-solving

State: Difficulties at work can be some of the most stressful problems confronting us. Think about the following situation. What could you do to manage it?

Take participants through the following scenario:

- What will you do/say to your supervisor?
- Role-play solutions to this situation using 'I' statements. Provide participants with the opportunity to share workplace experiences

22. Relaxation exercise

Take participants through the deep breathing relaxation exercise once again.

23. Finishing up

RECALL: Recapitulate what has been covered during the session:

- understanding the personal consequences of hearing loss;
- ways and ideas/strategies to improve communication and lifestyle;
- exercises in self assertion and relaxation;
- managing difficulties at work;
- finding out about available resources.

Personal contract

Objective

To enable participants to identify goals for change following the workshop.

MATERIALS: Provide participants with the handout for personal contracts.

TIME: 20–30 minutes.

Process

Present and explain the 'Personal contract'.

The workshop has given participants a chance to think about things like improving their communication, assertiveness and relaxation skills. Now comes the time for action. What things in your life do you think you can, or

Personal contract

From now until the next meeting I intend to:

- explain to people that I have a hearing problem
- make requests in keeping with my hearing problem
- investigate and/or get myself a new telephone with volume control
- investigate and/or get myself a TV aid
- investigate hearing aids
- investigate and/or get myself a cochlear implant/use my accessories
- investigate/get myself/use accessories that go with my cochlear implant speech processor
- look more at people when I'm listening to them
- Other (please say what)....................................
-
- Signed.................................
- Date..................................

Figure 10.24: Personal contract.

would like to, improve? The personal contract represents a commitment that you undertake to improve your situation in connection with your hearing problem.

- *Recall* that since the start of the workshop participants have become familiar with several ways of improving communication. Ask the participants to take a few minutes with their partners to discuss any changes they would like to adopt.
- Write on the handout 'Personal contract', the choice(s) made by each participant and their names (make a note of these choices on a piece of paper so they can be verified during the return meeting, three months later).

Follow-up workshop

Announce that they will be invited to return in three months in order to share with the rest of the group what they have done to improve communication in their lives since coming to the workshop. Fix an appropriate date for the coming meeting (three months). Inform them that you will tell them of the next meeting by mail or by telephone.

Evaluation of the workshop

Evaluate the session verbally by asking participants:

- What is the most important thing you have learnt from these sessions?
- What did you find the least useful?
- Do you believe that what you have learnt will help you in your everyday life?
- In what way has the presence of your partners changed anything in the way the workshop went?
- What made you decide to come to this meeting?
- Did your partner have something to do with your decision to come to this meeting?

Thank everyone for their participation in the group, noting that the success of the programme pivoted on their contributions.

Close

After having finished the session: Replace the equipment and the furniture in the room as required. In discussion with co-workers, revise the sessions:

What are your first impressions on:
- achieving the objectives of the sessions?
- the development of the group over the sessions?
- your roles as organizer?

- What were your strong points?
- What were the points needing improvements?
- What resources can you draw on for these improvements?
- In reorganizing this session, what would you do differently?

Establish ways of making improvements before the next programme.

The follow-up meeting – 3 months later

One month after the session, participants should be sent a letter of encouragement. The purpose of this letter is to maintain contact and to remind people that they have goals they need to be working on (see Figure 10.25: Sample letter).

Three months after the session, contact participants by telephone again and invite the people to a follow-up meeting. You should telephone

Sample follow-up letter

Hello everyone,
You will remember recently doing a workshop with me on living with Hearing Loss. At this meeting, as well as looking at the impact of hearing loss in our lives, we saw several ways to make life easier with our hearing problems.

For example, we saw that by planning ahead or being assertive, one could make hearing in difficult places more manageable. You will also have realized that there are non-technical means to help oneself, in particular, in group meetings or in outings. We all know the usual tactics for improving communication like asking people to talk more slowly, repeating, talking face to face, and reducing background noise. In the group the key to success was identified as being confident and assertive and being prepared to plan ahead to minimize the chance of problems arising. Through planning and being assertive we can make communicating easier and we can lessen stress by using relaxation.

It's been 3 months since we met and it's time for a brief follow-up meeting. The purpose of the meeting is to see where you are now, to find out what you've been doing and to see if there is anything else we can do to support you as you move on to manage your everyday communication needs. As well, we would like some feedback on what you thought of the workshop and how it can be improved.

Looking forward to seeing you again at (place, time, date)

Figure 10.25: Sample follow-up letter that may be used to invite participants to follow-up meeting.

roughly ten days before the actual meeting. You can remind them of the objectives of the last meeting:

1. Support them with their chosen plan of action.
2. Repeat information if necessary.
3. Evaluate the impact and the effects of the programme in their lives.

Objectives

Specify the objectives of the follow-up meeting:

- to see what has changed and what has happened since last time we met;
- to see if there are any other questions participants might have;
- to administer follow-up questionnaires if a formal evaluation is taking place.

TIME: 2 hours.

- Recall what happened last time the group met.
- Make a brief résumé of the last session (say 5 minutes).

PROCESS

Set up the FM system and make sure it is working well. Welcome the participants back again. Take people through an ice breaker exercise quickly.

Inform the participants of the approximate duration of the meeting.

Redo the birthday party exercise.

Workshop people thoroughly, recalling the principles of communication covered in previous sessions. This activity will take place separately between the people with hearing loss and partners.

FOR THE PEOPLE WITH HEARING LOSS:

Remain in the meeting place with one group leader. Pose the following questions:

In the family:

- What are you doing differently?
- Do you see yourself differently?
- Do you feel different?

In social activities:

- What are you doing differently?
- Do you see yourself differently?
- Do you feel different?

At work:

- What are you doing differently?
- Do you see yourself differently?
- Do you feel different?

For the partners:

In another room, a group leader interviews the partners.

In the family:

- What are they doing differently?
- Do they see themselves differently?
- Do they feel different?

At social activities:

- What are they doing differently?
- Do they see themselves differently?
- Do they feel different?

As a group:

- Reunite all the participants and bring out the comments that people with hearing loss and partners made.

Relaxation:

- Question the participants to find out if they followed up on the relaxation exercises.
- If yes – did the exercises help them to live with less stress?
- If no, why not? What else could be done to help?

Hearing Help Cards:

- Did they use the Hearing Help Cards?
- If yes: Where? When? How did people react?

Relevance of meetings:

- Verify with them whether the fact of organizing meetings as a group is a good way of doing communication training and confidence building.
- What did they find most useful about coming to these meetings?
- What was the least important, the least helpful for them, from all that they have seen and done?

Closing the meeting:

- Thank participants for their attendance and participation.
- Tell them that they can get in touch with you if they need information or help.

Appendix: Methodological issues

The qualitative data reported in this text study is based upon the principles of a descriptive evaluation design that utilizes a case study method as the central research and analytical tool. The design is non-experimental, inductive and qualitative. Twenty-one semi-structured interviews were conducted with deafened adults with cochlear implants and family members from around Australia. Participants were initially recruited by a process of random selection and postal recruitment (15 people); the remainder were consequently recruited by a process of snowballing (respondent or peer-identified participants). Random selection was used to facilitate a systematic point of entry into the field as it provided a straightforward way of ensuring that participants from each state in Australia had the opportunity to participate in the study. It was not used as a tool for generating a sample in order to make statistical generalizations about the population of people with cochlear implants. The structure of interviews centred on the integration of the theorised life-history method (Plummer, 1987) within Foucault's philosophical framework of technologies of the self (Foucault, 1988).

Plummer (1987) observes that within the life-history method, 'the researcher is merely there in the first instance to give "voice" to other people; in some circumstances the voices may be interpreted'. In consequence, the presentation of the research material is structured within a narrative format that presents the experiences of people who engage in a technology-focused process of hearing rehabilitation with a view to remaking themselves as a hearing person. This narrative is further developed by considering the issues confronting respondents in the light of one of the guiding principles underpinning sociological research:

> many personal troubles cannot be merely solved as troubles, but must be understood in terms of public issues (Mills, 1970).

Interviews were recorded on audiotape and subsequently transcribed. Interviews were subjected to a reflexive process of analysis that moved between content analysis of themes arising within the text and the literature that informed the research. Each interview was written up in the style of a personal narrative. The narrative developed the themes arising from the interview and integrated these with the theoretical frameworks informing the study. The purpose of this analytical approach was to bring out the key issues that concerned individuals, to draw attention to what it was they were trying to achieve, not just with a cochlear implant, but within their lives generally. As Dowsett (1996: 55) observes,

> the key to the theorized life-history method is its intent, the explication of social process, not biography. It is important to make no special effort to avoid paradox, contradiction or inconsistency. There should be no 'papering over the cracks', but an embracing of discontinuity and ambiguity within a subject's life.

In consequence, enduring inconsistencies in themes were subjected to Gerson's (1989) procedure for supplementing grounded theory which utilizes inconsistencies as a strategy for better understanding the theoretical issues under examination. In such cases the question is posed: does the exception prove the rule?

Excerpts from these interviews appear in the text under the names of Jean, Rick, Liz, Jack, Dominic, Gena, Sandra, Christine, Jan, Jeff, Paul, Ellen, Roger, Carol, Fiona and Paula. These people are Deafened adults with implants. In some instances, gender and other identifiers have been changed to protect respondent privacy.

Quantitative data reported in Chapter 4 was collected as a part of a cross-sectional study of audiologists' attitudes to cochlear implants and tactile aids. One third of audiologists working in Australia responded to the study. The questionnaire used was developed by the Battelle Institute, Virginia, and was made available to me courtesy of Cochlear Ltd. The full paper on audiologists' attitudes to cochlear implants was published in Cochlear Implants International Volume 2:2 2001. Quantitative psychosocial data reported in Chapter 7 was collected from 129 implantees who participated in a cross-sectional survey associated with my PhD studies. For further details see Hogan, 1997. A psychosocial survey was also completed by 202 deafened adults with cochlear implants in Australia and New Zealand in 1998/99, 148 of whom had cochlear implants (Hogan et al., 2000) Within this survey, respondents were asked to report their occupation, education and employment status. These details were reported in Chapter 2.

References

Abberley P (1993) Disabled people and 'normality'. In J Swain, V Finkelstein, S French, M Oliver (eds) Disabling Barriers – Enabling Environments. London: Sage Publications, 107–15.

Anderson M (1991) Services for hearing impaired people and training for health workers in Denmark. Auration, No. 1, National Acoustic Laboratory, Chatwoods, Australia.

Andreas C, Andreas T (1994) Core Transformation: Reaching the Wellspring Within. Utah, USA: Real People Press.

Asher SR, Wheeler VA (1993) Children's loneliness: a comparison of rejected and neglected children. Journal of Consulting and Clinical Psychology 53, 500–5, cited in N Weinberg, M Sterritt (1991) Disability and identity: a study of identity patterns in adolescents with hearing impairments. In MG Eisenberg, RL Glueckauf (eds), Empirical Approaches to the Psychosocial Aspects of Disability. New York: Springer, 68–84.

Australian Bureau of Statistics (1993a) Disability, Ageing and Carers – Hearing Impairment. Catalogue No. 4435.0. Canberra: Australian Government Printing Service.

Australian Bureau of Statistics (1993b) Disability, Ageing and Carers – Summary of findings. Catalogue No. 4430.0. Canberra: Australian Government Printing Service.

Australian Bureau of Statistics (1993c) Labor Force Status and Educational Attainment – February. Catalogue No. 6205.0. Canberra: Australian Government Printing Service.

Australian Bureau of Statistics (1995). Labor Force of Australia – June. Total person 15 years and older Catalogue No. 6203.0. Canberra: Australian Government Printing Service.

Australian Bureau of Statistics (1998) Labour Force. Catalogue 6203.0. Canberra: Australian Government Printing Service.

Australian Bureau of Statistics (1999) Year Book. Canberra: Australian Government Printing Service.

Baron RA, Byrne D (1987) Social Psychology: Understanding Human Interaction, 5th edn. Sydney: Allyan & Bacon.

Bauman Z (1995) Life in Fragments: Essays in Postmodern Morality. Oxford: Blackwell.

Beck U (1992) Risk Society: Towards a New Modernity. London: Sage Publications.

Bell AG (1917) The growth of the oral method in America. Paper presented at the 50th anniversary of the founding of the Clarke School, Northampton, MA. 10 October 1917. Library. Volta Bureau, Washington DC.

Bender R (1970) The Conquest of Deafness: A History of the Long Struggles to Make Possible Normal Living to Those Handicapped by Lack of Normal Hearing. Cleveland, OH: The Press of Case Western Reserve University.

Bolton R (1987) People Skills: How to Asset Yourself, Listen to Others and Resolve Conflicts. Australia. Simon & Schuster.

Bourdieu P (1977) Outline of a Theory of Practice. Cambridge: Cambridge University Press.

Bourdieu P (1990) The Logic of Practice. Cambridge: Polity Press.

Bourdieu P (1992) Thinking about limits. Theory, Culture and Society 9(1), February: 37–50.

Breuig HL (1990) The legacy of Dr. Bell. The Volta Review 92(4): 83–96.

Brooks S (1994) Rehabilitation for adults cochlear implantees. A presentation paper covering rehabilitation for post-lingual adult cochlear implantees. Lane Cove, Sydney: Cochlear Pty Ltd, October.

Burchell G, Gordon C, Miller P (eds) (1991) The Foucault Effect. London: Harvester Wheatsheaf.

Carlson JG, Hatfield E (1992) Psychology of Emotion. Sydney: Harcourt Brace Jovanovic College Publishers.

Carter R, Hailey D (1995) Economic evaluation of the cochlear implant. Centre for Health Programme Evaluation. Working paper 44. Melbourne.

Charmaz K (1990) 'Discovering' chronic illness: using grounded theory. Social Science and Medicine 30(11): 1161–72.

Clark GM (1997) Cochlear implants. XVI World Congress of Otorhinolaryngology Head and Neck Surgery, Sydney, 2–7 March 1997, Monduzzi Editore International Proceedings Division Bologna.

Clark GM, Cowan R (1995) (eds) International Cochlear Implant, Speech and Hearing Symposium – Melbourne 1994. Annals of Otology, Rhinology and Laryngology Supplement 166, Vol. 104(9), Part 2: 201–6.

Clark GM, Blamey PJ, Brown AM, Gusby PA, Dowell RC, Franz BK-H, Pyman BC, Shepherd YC, Tong YC, Webb RL, Hirshorn MS, Kuzma J, Mecklenberg DJ, Money DK, Patrick JF, Seligman PM (1987) The University of Melbourne: nucleus multi-electrode cochlear implant. In CR Pfaltz (ed.), Advances in Oto-Rhino-Laryngology, Vol. 38, 1–18.

Clark GM, Shepherd RK, Franz BK-H et al. (1988) The biologic safety of the cochlear corporation multiple-electrode intracochlear implant. American Journal of Otology 9(1): 8–13.

Clark GM, Cohen NL, Shepherd RK (1991a) Surgical and safety considerations of multi-channel cochlear implants. Ear and Hearing 12(4), Supplement: 15s–24s.

Clark GM, Dowell RC, Pyman BC et al. (1991b) Clinical trial of a multi-channel cochlear prosthesis: results on 10 post-lingually deaf patients. Australian and New Zealand Journal of Surgery 54(6), December: 519–26.

Code C, Müller DJ (1992) Code–Müller Protocol: Assessing Perceptions of Psychosocial Adjustment to Aphasia and Related Disorders. London: Whurr.

Code C, Khanbha F, Mattiazzo V (1996) Perceptions of emotional and psychosocial state in laryngectomised patients, their significant others and speech pathologists. Disability and Rehabilitation 18(11): 567–84.

Cohen K (1992) Taoist Healing Imagery – Traditional Chinese Healing Visualization (audiotape). Boulder, CO: Sounds True Production.

Cole SH, Edelman RJ (1991) Identity patterns and self- and teacher-perceptions of problems for deaf adolescents, a research note. Journal of Child Psychology, Psychiatry and Allied Health Professions 32(7): 1159–65.

Cordell J (1978) Early History of National Acoustic Laboratories, Internal Report No 6, National Acoustic Laboratories. Millers Point, Sydney: Australian Department of Health.

Corker M (1998) Deaf and Disabled or Deafness Disabled. Buckingham: Open University Press.

Coryell J, Holcomb TK, Scherer M (1992) Attitudes toward deafness: a collegiate perspective. American Annals of the Deaf 137(3): 299–302.

Davis A, Wood S (1992) The epidemiology of childhood hearing impairment, factors relevant to planning services. British Journal of Audiology 26: 77–90.

Davis LJ (1995) Enforcing Normalcy – Disability, Deafness and the Body. London: Verso.

De Saint-Loup A. (1993) Images of the deaf in medieval western Europe. In R Fischer, H Lane (eds), Looking Back: A Reader on the History of Deaf Communities and their Sign Languages. Hamburg: Signum Press, 379–402.

Dean M (1991) The Constitution of Poverty: Toward a Genealogy of Liberal Governance. London: Routledge.

Dean M (1992) A genealogy of the government of poverty. Economy and Society 21(3), August, 215–251.

Dean M (1994) 'A social structure of many souls': moral regulation, government and self-formation. Canadian Journal of Sociology 19(2): 145–68.

Diprose R (1993) Nietzsche and the pathos of distance. In P Patton (ed.), Nietzsche, Feminism and Political Thought. Sydney: Allen & Unwin, 9–26.

Dowsett GW (1994) Sexual Contexts and Homosexually Active Men in Australia. Canberra: Commonwealth Department of Human Services and Health, Australian Government Publishing Service.

Dowsett GW (1996) Homosexual Desire. Stanford, CA: Stanford University Press.

Draper P (1992) Quality of life as quality of being, an alternative to the subject–object dichotomy. Journal of Advanced Nursing 17: 965–70.

Drummond M (1987) Methods for the Economic Evaluation of Health Care. Oxford: Oxford University Press.

Durant J (1986) The ascent of nature in the ascent of man. In D Kohn, Darwinian Heritage. Princeton, NJ: Princeton University Press, 283–306.

Durkheim E (1971) On social facts. In M Truzzi (1971) Sociology: The Classic Statements. New York: Random House, 55–64.

Edwards M (1994) Deafness and Hearing Impairment in Ancient Greece. Unpublished PhD thesis, Minneapolis, USA: University of Minnesota Press, 1–34.

Egan G (1975) The Skilled Helper: Model, Skills and Methods For Effective Helping. Monterey, CA: Brooks/Cole.

Eisenwort B, Brauenis K, Burian K (1985) Rehabilitation of the cochlear implant patient. In RF Gray, Cochlear Implants. London: Croom, Helm and College-Hill Press Inc..

Epstein J (1989) The Story of the Bionic Ear. Melbourne: Hyland Publishing House.

Erber NP (1988) Communication Therapy for Hearing-Impaired Adults. Victoria: Clavis Publishing.

Erickson EH (1965) Childhood and Society. Harmondsworth: Penguin.

Finkelstein V (1980) Attitudes and Disabled People. New York: World Rehabilitation Fund.

Foucault M (1963) The Birth of the Clinic: An Archaeology of Medical Perception. London: Routledge.

Foucault M (1977, 1979) Discipline and Punish: The Birth of the Prison. New York: Vintage Books.

Foucault M (1980) Power and Knowledge: Selected interviews and other writings 1972–1977, ed. C Gordon. New York: Harvester Wheatsheaf.

Foucault M (1988) Technologies of the self. In LH Martin, H Gutman, PH Hutton (eds), Technologies of the Self: A Seminar with Michel Foucault. London: Tavistock, 16–49.

Foucault M (1989) Résumé des cours. Paris: Juillard.

Foucault M (1990) The Use of Pleasure: The History of Sexuality, Volume 2. USA: Vintage Books.

Foucault M (1991a) Governmentality. In G Burchell, C Gordon, P Miller (eds), The Foucault Effect: Studies in Governmentality. London: Harvester Wheatsheaf, 87–104.

Foucault M (1991b) Politics and the study of discourse. In G Burchell, C Gordon, P Miller (eds), The Foucault Effect: Studies in Governmentality. London: Harvester Wheatsheaf, 53–72.

Foucault M (1991c) Questions of method. In G Burchell, C Gordon, P Miller (eds), The Foucault Effect: Studies in Governmentality. London: Harvester Wheatsheaf, 73–86.

Foucault M (1991d, 1963) The Birth of the Clinic – An Archaeology of Medical Perception. London: Routledge.

Foucault M (1992) Orders of discourse. In S Lash (ed.), Post-structuralist and Post-Modernist Sociology. An Elgar Reference Collection, University of Lancaster.

Fulcher G (1989) Disabling policies? A Comparative Approach to Education Policy and Disability. London: Falmer Press.

Fulcher G (1992a) Picking up the pieces! What do recreation workers need to know about policy and working with people with severe disabilities? Melbourne: Department of Leisure and Tourism, Phillip Institute of Technology. Manuscript 121 pp.

Fulcher G (1992b) Pigs' tails and peer workers: the view from Victoria, Australia. In L Barton, Disability and the Necessity for a Socio-political Perspective. The International Exchange of Experts and Information in Rehabilitation. National Institute of Disability and Rehabilitation Research, World Rehabilitation Fund, University of New Hampshire Press, Durham, USA, 23–34.

Fulcher G (1993) Modern identity and severe disability: How might recreation workers encourage people with severe disabilities to live? Towards a framework. Melbourne: Department of Leisure and Tourism, Royal Melbourne Institute of Technology. Manuscript 86 pp.

Fulcher G (1996) Beyond normalization but not utopia. In L Barton (ed.) Disability and Society: Emerging Issues and Insights. London: Longman.

Fusfeld DR (1994) The Age of the Economist, 7th edn. New York: HarperCollins College Publishers.

Gaeth JH (1979) A history of aural rehabilitation. In MA Henoch (ed.), Aural Rehabilitation for the Elderly. New York: Grune & Stratton, 1–21.

Gerson EM (1989) Supplementing grounded theory. In D Maines (ed.), Social Organisation and Social Process: Essays in Honor of Anselm Strauss. New York: Aldine de Gruyter, 285–301.

Getty L, Hetu R (1991) Development of a rehabilitation programme for people affected with occupational hearing loss. 2. Results from group intervention with 48 workers and their spouses, Audiology 30: 317–29.

Giddens A (1991) Modernity and Self-identity. Self and Society in the Late Modern Age. Cambridge: Polity Press.

Goffman I (1963) Stigma. London: Penguin.

Goffman I (1973) The Presentation of Self in Everyday Life. New York: Overlook Press.

Gordon C (1991) Governmental rationality: an introduction. In G Burchell, C Gordon, P Miller (eds), The Foucault Effect: Studies in Governmentality. London: Harvester Wheatsheaf, 1–52.

Habermas J (1990) Moral Consciousness and Communicative Action. Cambridge: Polity Press.

Hawe P, Degeling D, Hall J (1990) Evaluating Health Promotion: A Health Worker's Guide. Sydney: MacLennan & Petty.

Hawthorne G, Richardson J, Osborne R (1999) The Assessment of Quality of Life (AQoL) Instrument: a psychometric measure of health related quality of life. Quality of Life Research 8: 209–44

Hemsley G, Code C (1996) Interactions between recovery in aphasia, emotional and psychosocial factors in subjects with aphasia, their significant others and speech pathologists. Disability and Rehabilitation 18: 567–84.

Henoch MA (1979) (ed.) Aural Rehabilitation for the Elderly. New York: Grune & Stratton.

Herrmann M, Wallesch CW (1989) Psychosocial changes and adjustment with chronic aphasic patient and family. Allied Health and Behavioural Sciences 2: 273–86.

Herrmann M, Wallesch CW (1990) Expectations of psychosocial adjustment in aphasia: a MAUT study with the Code-Müller Scale of Psychosocial Adjustment. Aphasiology 4: 527–38.

Herrmann M, Code C (1996) Weightings of items on the Code-Müller-Protocols: the effects of clinical experience on aphasia therapy. Disability and Rehabilitation 18: 509–14.

Hetu R, Getty L (1991) Development of a rehabilitation programme for people affected with occupational hearing loss. 1. A new paradigm. Audiology, 305–16.

Hogan A (1991a) Rehabilitation for workers suffering noise–induced hearing loss. Australian and New Zealand Journal of Occupational Health and Safety 7(1): 35–42.

Hogan A (1991b) 'Setting the Agenda' Redefining: The Experiences of Some Young Deaf Men. 2nd International Conference; European Society for Deafness and Mental Health, 9–11 May, Belgium: La Bastide.

Hogan A (1992a) Communication competencies for working with people with hearing loss. Cumberland Hearing Rehabilitation and Research Centre, University of Sydney.

Hogan A (1992b) Rehabilitation for workers with noise-induced hearing loss – a community health approach. Master of Science thesis. University of Wollongong, Australia.

Hogan A (1995a) People with acquired hearing loss A submission to the Commonwealth, State, Disability Review. Burwood, Sydney: Woodstock Community Centre.

Hogan A (1995b) The governance of deafened adults. Society for Disability Studies Conference proceedings, San Francisco, CA.

Hogan A (1996) A cochlear odyssey. PhD thesis, Macquarie University, Sydney.

Hogan A (1997) Implant outcomes – towards a mixed methodology for evaluating the efficacy of adult cochlear implant programmes. Disability and Rehabilitation 19(6): 233–44; 793–805.

Hogan A (1998a) The business of hearing. Health 2(4): 485–501.

Hogan A (1998b) Carving out a space to act – acquired impairment and contested identity, Health 2(1): 75–90.

Hogan A, Brown K, Brown M, Smith B (1989) Project Knock! Knock! A profile of the Deaf Community of New South Wales. Sydney: Deaf Society of New South Wales.

Hogan A, Ewan C, Noble W, Munnerley G (1994) Coping with occupational hearing loss. An application in Australia of the University of Montreal Acoustics Group Rehabilitation Programme. Australian and New Zealand Journal of Occupational Health and Safety 10(2): 107–18.

Hogan A, Taylor A, Code C (1999) Employment outcomes for people with cochlear implants. Australian Journal of Rehabilitation Counselling 5(1): 1–8.

Hogan A, Hawthorne G, Taylor A, Code C (2000) Quality of life outcomes for people with cochlear implants, poster abstract, CI2000, Loews Miami Beach Hotel, Miami, FL, February.

Hollon SD, Kendall PC (1980) Cognitive self statements in depression: development of an automatic thoughts questionnaire. Cognitive Therapy and Research 4(4): 383–95.

Hollows R, Dowell RC, Cowan RSC, Skok MC, Pyman BC, Clark GM (1995) Continuing improvements in speech processing for adult cochlear implant patients. In GM Clark, R Cowan (eds), International Cochlear Implant, Speech and Hearing Symposium – Melbourne 1994. Annals of Otology, Rhinology and Laryngology Supplement 166, Vol. 104(9), Part 2: 292–4.

Horney K (1959) The basic conflict. In L Gorlow, W Katkovsky (eds), Readings in the Psychology of Adjustment. New York: McGraw Hill.

Jagose A (1993) Slash and suture: post/colonialism in 'Borderland/La Frontera: The New Mestiza'. In S Gunew, A Yeatman (eds) Feminism and the Politics of Difference. Sydney: Allen & Unwin, 212–27.

Jones L, Kyle J, Wood PL (1987) Words Apart: Losing Your Hearing as an Adult. London: Tavistock.

Jung C (1983) The Essential Jung. Selected and introduced by Anthony Storr. London: Fontana Press, HarperCollins.

Kaplan H, Bally SJ, Garretson C (1985) Speechreading: A Way to Improve Understanding. Washington, DC: Gallaudet College Press.

Knutson JF, Schartz HA, Gantz BJ (1991a) Psychological change following 18 months of cochlear implant use. Annals of Otology, Rhinology and Laryngology 100(11), Nov: 877–82.

Knutson JF, Hinrichs JV, Tyler RS (1991b) Psychological predictors of audiological outcomes of multichannel cochlear implants, preliminary findings. Annals of Otology, Rhinology and Laryngology 100(10), Oct: 817–22.

Lane H (1979) The Wild Boy of Aveyron. Cambridge, MA: Harvard University Press.

Lane H (1984) When the Mind Hears a History of the Deaf. New York: Random House.

Lane H (1993) The Mask of Benevolence Disabling the Deaf Community. New York: Vintage Books, Random House.

Lash S (1990) Postmodernism as humanism? Urban space and social theory. In BS Turner (ed.), Theories of Modernity and Postmodernity. London: Sage Publications.

Lash S (1991) Genealogy and the body, Foucault/Deleuze/Nietzsche. In M Featherstone, M Hepworth, BS Turner (eds), The Body, Social Process and Cultural Theory. London: Sage Publications, 256–80.

Laws J (ed.) (1991) A Sociology of Monsters. London: Routledge.

Lutman ME, Brown EJ, Coles RRA (1987). Self-reported disability and handicap in the population in relation to pure-tone threshold, age, sex and type of hearing loss. British Journal of Audiology 21: 45–58.

Luxford WM, Brackman DE (1985) The history of cochlear implants. In RF Gray (ed.), Cochlear Implants. Sydney: Croon Helm, 1–26.

Mergler D (1987) Worker participation in occupational health research: theory and practice. International Journal of Health Services 17(1).

Mills CW (1970) The sociological imagination. Harmondsworth: Penguin.

Minichiello V, Aroni R, Timewell E et al. (1990) In-depth Interviewing Researching People. Australia: Longman Chesire.

Moore H (1994) A Passion for Difference. Cambridge: Polity Press.

Noble WG (1991) Why is hearing impairment so handicapping. In Occupational Noise-induced Hearing Loss Rehabilitation and Prevention. Sydney:University of New England, Armidale and Worksafe Australia.

Noble WG, Hetu R (1994) An ecological approach to disability and handicaps in relation to hearing impairment. Audiology 33(2), March–April: 117–26.

Oliver M (1990) The Politics of Disablement. London: Macmillan,.

Oliver M (1993a) Disability and dependency: a creation of industrial societies. In J Swain, V Finkelstein, S French, M Oliver (eds), Disabling Barriers: Enabling Environments. London: Sage Publications, 49–60.

Oliver M (1993b) Re-defining disability: a challenge to research. In J Swain, V Finkelstein, S French, M Oliver (eds), Disabling Barriers: Enabling Environments. London: Sage Publications, 61–8.

Oliver M (1996) Understanding Disability: From Theory to Practice. London: Macmillan.

Oliver M, Zarb G, Silver J, Moore M, Salisbury V (1988) Walking into Darkness: The Experience of Spinal Cord Injury. London: Macmillan Press.

Orlans H (1988) Confronting deafness in an unstilled world. Society 25(4), May/June: 32–9.

Parsons T (1951) The Social System. New York: Free Press.

Pengilley P (1975) Aural Rehabilitation: Churchill Fellowship Report. Jolimont, Australia: Vctorian Hear Service.

Pfeiffer D (1994) Eugenics and disability discrimination. Disability and Society 9(4): 481–99.

Pfeiffer D (1995) The international classification of impairment, disability and handicap. Paper presented at the 8th Annual Meeting, Society for Disability Studies, Parc Oakland Hotel, Oakland, CA. 15–19 June. Manuscript 34 pp.

Plant G (1976) Aural rehabilitation programmes for deafened adults. Australian Journal of Human Communication Disorders 4(1), June.

Plant G (1977) Adult Aural Rehabilitation: A Report on World Health Organisation Fellowship. Sydney: National Acoustic Laboratory.

Plummer K (1987) Documents of Life: An Introduction to the Problems and Literature of a Humanistic Method. London: George, Allen & Unwin.

Reed V, Hogan A, Munnerley G, Lee K (1994) Adults with acquired hearing loss: identification and referral patterns of community health workers. Australian Journal of Public Health 18(2): 223–5.

Rutman D (1989) The impact and experience of adventitious deafness. American Annals of the Deaf 134(4), December: 305–10.

Sacks O (1989) Seeing Voices. London: Picador.

Sawicki J (1991) Disciplining Foucault. New York: Routledge, Chapman & Hall.

Sherbourne K, White L (1997) An Evaluation of the Impact of Rehabilitation Courses for Deafened Adults run by the Link Centre for Deafened People. Manuscript.

Silverman D (1989) Telling convincing stories: a plea for cautious positivism in case studies. In B Glassner, JD Moreni (eds.), The Qualitative-Quantitative Distinction in the Social Sciences. Dordrecht: Kluwer, 57–77.

Spencer PE (2000) The Deaf Child in the Family and at School: Essays in honor of Kathryn P. Meadows-Orlans. Erlbaum, New Jersey: Lawrence Erlbaum Associates.

Starr SL (1991) Power, technologies and the phenomenology of conventions, on being allergic to onions. In J Laws (ed.), A Sociology of Monsters. London: Routledge, 26–56.

Summerfield Q, Marshall DH (1995) Pre-operative predictors of outcomes from cochlear implantation in adults: performance and quality of life. In GM Clark, R Cowan (eds.), International Cochlear Implant, Speech and Hearing Symposium – Melbourne 1994. Annals of Otology, Rhinology and Laryngology, Supplement 166, Vol. 104(9), Part 2: 105–8.

Summerfield Q, Marshall DH, Davis AC (1995) Cochlear implantation: demand, costs and utility. In GM Clark, R Cowan (eds), International Cochlear Implant, Speech and Hearing Symposium – Melbourne 1994. Annals of Otology, Rhinology and Laryngology, Supplement 166, vol. 104(9), Part 2: 245–8.

Swain J, Finkelstein V, French S, Oliver M (eds) (1993) Disabling Barriers: Enabling Environments. London: Sage Publications.

Taylor A, Dal Grande E, Cooper J, Wilson D, Manser T (1999) The South Australian Survey of Disability Prevalence: November 1996–February 1997. Hindmarsh Sq, Adelaide: SERCIS, Behavioural Epidemiology Unit, Epidemiology Branch, South Australian Health Commission.

Thomas A (1981) Acquired deafness and mental health. British Journal of Medical Psychology 54: 219–29.

Warren M (1988) Nietzsche and Political Thought. Cambridge, MA: MIT Press.

Weinberg N, Sterritt M (1991) Disability and identity: a study of identity patterns in adolescents with hearing impairments. In MG Eisenberg, RL Glueckauf (eds),

Empirical Approaches to the Psychosocial Aspects of Disability. New York: Springer Publishing Company.

Westcott S, Kato J (1998) 'Living with Deafness': a residential workshop to improve communication for deafened clients and partners. 13th Annual Conference, Novotel, Sydney: Australian Audiological Society.

Wilson D (1994) Hearing loss and diagnosis for the South Australian population, Hearing Priorities Towards 2000. Better Hearing Australia 48th Annual Conference, Adelaide, 7–11 August.

Wilson D (1997) Disability and Handicap: Hearing Loss in South Australia. PhD thesis, School of Medicine, University of Adelaide.

Wilson DH, Xibin S, Read P, Walsh P, Esterman A (1992) Hearing loss – an underestimated public health problem. Australian Journal of Public Health 16: 282–6.

Wilson DH, Taylor AW, Walsh PG et al. (1999) Epidemiology of hearing impairment in an Australian adult population. International Journal of Epidemiology 28(2): 247–52.

Windmill IM, Martinez SA, Nolph MB, Eisenmenger BA (1990) Surgical and nonsurgical complications associated with cochlear prosthesis implantation. American Journal of Otology 11(6) , November: 415–20.

Winefield R (1987) Never the Twain Shall Meet: The Communications Debate. Washington, DC: Gallaudet University Press.

Winzer MA (1993) Education, urbanization, and the Deaf community: a case study of Toronto, 1870–1900. In J Vickey Van Cleve (ed.), Deaf History Unveiled: Interpretations from the New Scholarship. Washington, DC: Gallaudet University Press, 127–45.

Wolley M (1993) Acquired hearing loss; acquired oppression. In J Swain, V Finkelstein, S French, M Oliver (eds), Disabling Barriers – Enabling Environments. London: Sage Publications, 78–84.

Part IV
Handouts

(These sheets may be photocopied)

Rules for the workshop.

1. **Right to Pass** – while we would encourage you to participate and we value your contribution, it is important that you have the right to choose to participate or to pass. Passing means that you do not have to answer a question if you do not want to.
2. **Mutual Respect** – while you may not always agree with others' views/opinions, it is important to acknowledge them. When giving any feedback, try and give it descriptively rather than judgementally.
3. **One at a Time** – not talking over one another ➠ turn-taking. We have a range of hearing abilities in our group; that is, some people hear better than others, so therefore it is very important that only one person speaks at a time.
4. **Confidentiality** – while you can discuss what you've gained and learned from the workshop outside the group, it is important not to refer to people specifically by name. This is important so that people feel safe in expressing ideas and feelings.
5. **I Statements** – speaking for yourself ➠ owning feelings and ideas
6. **Finishing up** – sometimes the group may go off on tangents and we need to agree on a signal we can use which signifies that we need to wind things up. If this sign is made to you then it is time to finish up what you are saying so that we can move on.

Key difficulties

- Cocktail effect - can't distinguish sounds
- Like words tend to sound the same
- It's just harder to hear now
- Some loud sounds hurt my hearing
- Ringing or buzzing sounds in the ear

- Can’t hear TV/Radio
- Can’t hear on the ‘phone
- Can’t hear in group settings
- Can’t manage difficult situations
- Loss of confidence
- Tinnitus

Layout of the barbecue party

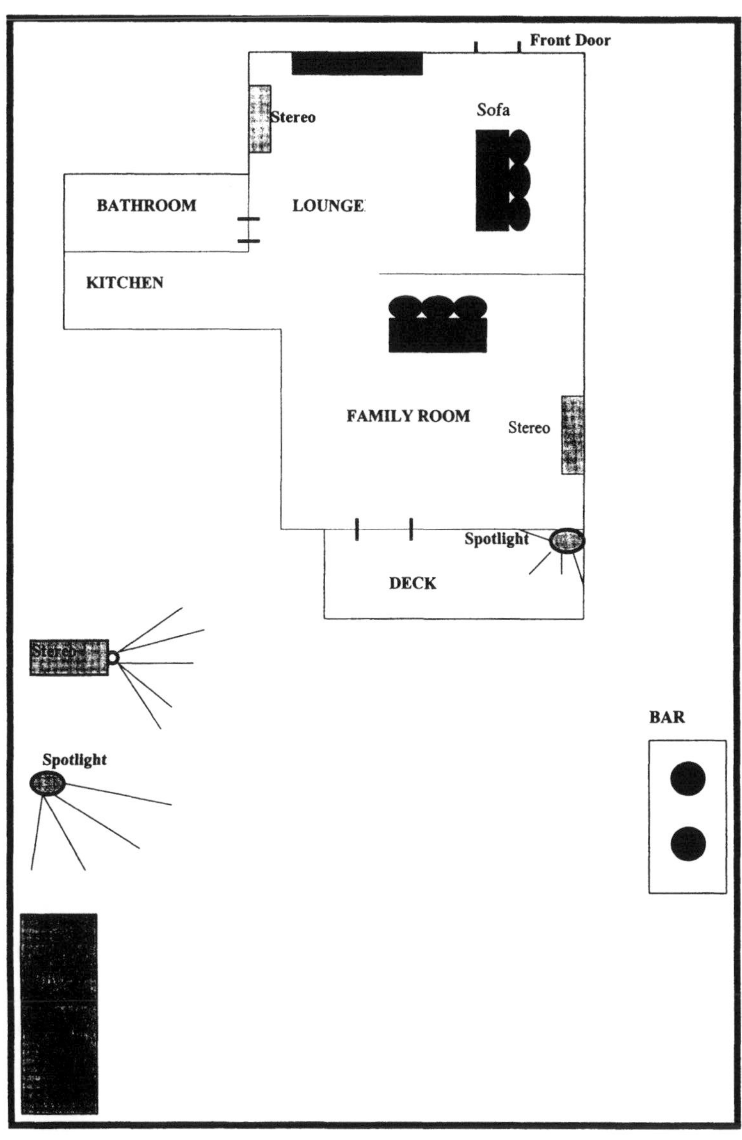

Barbecue birthday party handout for people with hearing loss

- Ann, your sister-in-law, has organized a big barbecue party for your brother's birthday. She has invited you, your partner and also some friends. When you arrive at their home you realize that there are about twenty people present and you do not know many of them. To create a real party atmosphere, for the evening, Ann has installed big outdoor candles all around the backyard and some loud speakers so that people can dance to the music. The food is excellent and the beer very good, people seem to really be enjoying themselves. It is becoming a little loud, it seems that everyone is talking at the same time and because a few people drink a little too much, their speech is more slurred. On top of that, in all the commotion you seem to have lost your partner. You realize that alone it is difficult to follow a conversation, you really did not understand the last joke someone just told. It looked very funny because everybody was laughing.

Barbecue birthday party handout for partners

- Ann, your sister-in-law, has organized a big barbecue party for your brother's birthday. She has invited you, your partner and also some friends. When you arrive at their home you realize that there are about twenty people present and you do not know many of them. To create a real party atmosphere, for the evening, Ann has installed big outdoor candles all around the backyard and some loud speakers so that people can dance to the music. The food is excellent and the beer very good, people seem to really be enjoying themselves. It is becoming a little loud, it seems that everyone is talking at the same time and because a few people drink a little too much, their speech is more slurred. You have found yourself chatting to a group away from your partner. You look over and realize that alone your partner is finding it difficult to follow the conversation; your partner clearly missed a joke that was just told. It looked very funny because everybody was laughing.

Strategies which help when talking to people

- Maintain visual contact
- Hold an upright posture
- Begin your sentences with 'I'
- Use short sentences and only say important things
- Try to remain relaxed

Strategies for dealing with difficult situations

- Eliminate the problem
- Assert your needs
- Negotiate a better communication environment
- Reduce noise/improve lighting,etc.
- Situate yourself away from the noise
- Put up with the problem
- Leave early/ go home/stay home

Common problems reported by partners

- Feeling guilty/frustrated
- Conflict management due to hearing loss
- Having to repeat
- Feeling ‘yelled’ at
- Noise from TV, etc.

Suggested layouts for stress exercise

Getting angry

Headaches

High pulse rate

Constipation

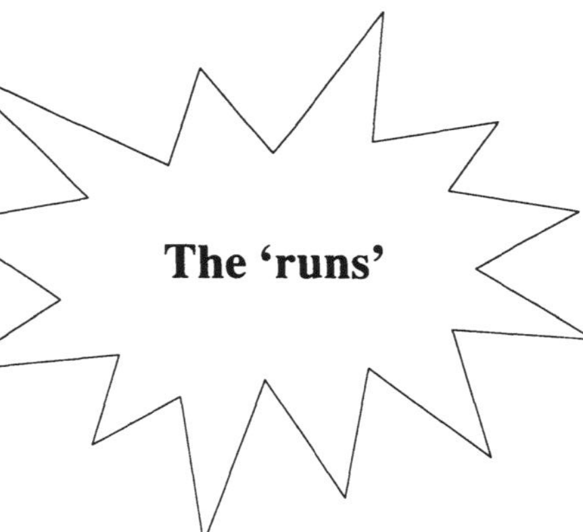
The 'runs'

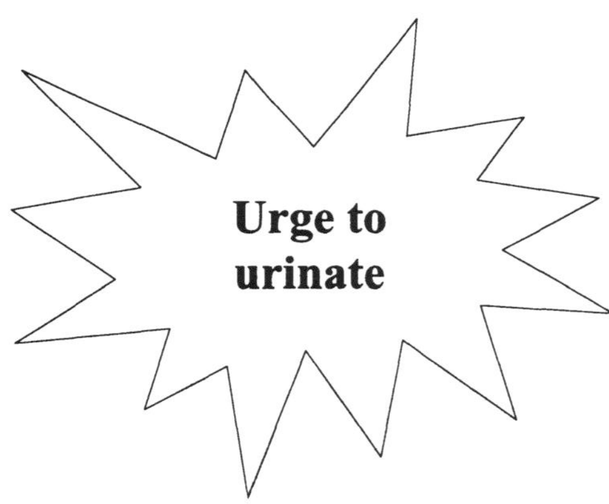
Urge to
urinate

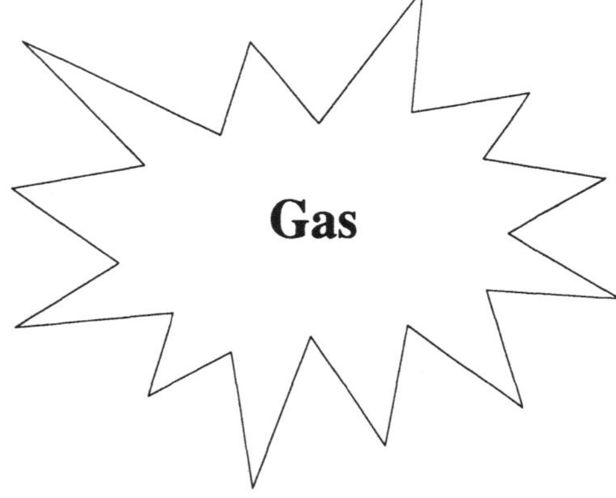
Gas

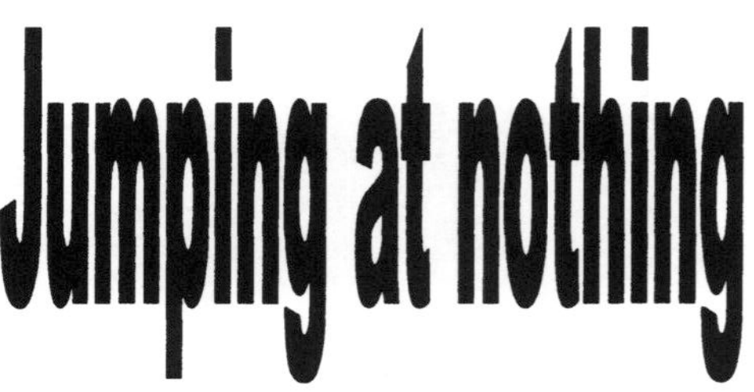
Jumping at nothing

Worrying

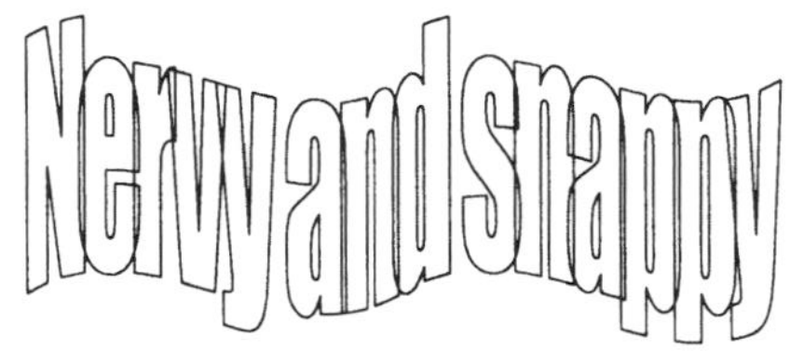

Constantly
on edge

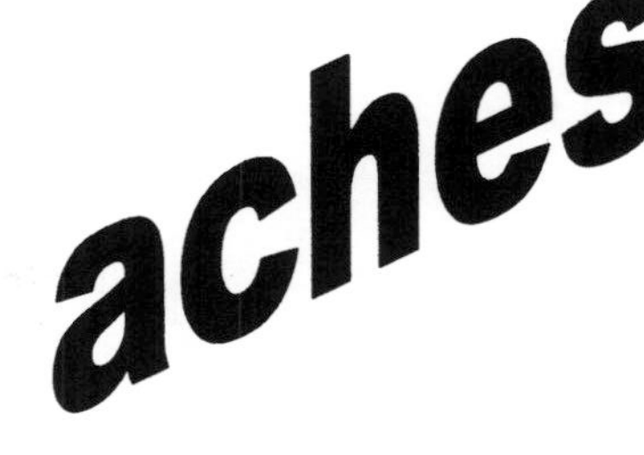

muscle tension

stiffness

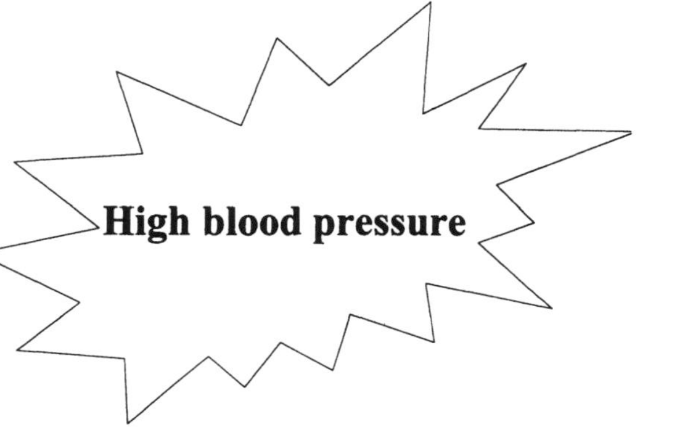

Depression

less agreeable life

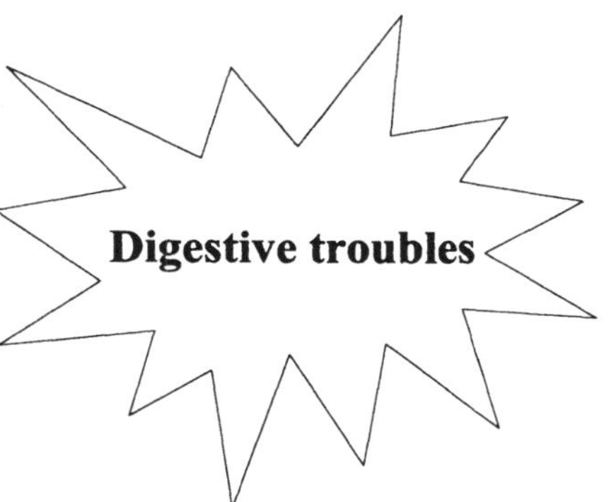

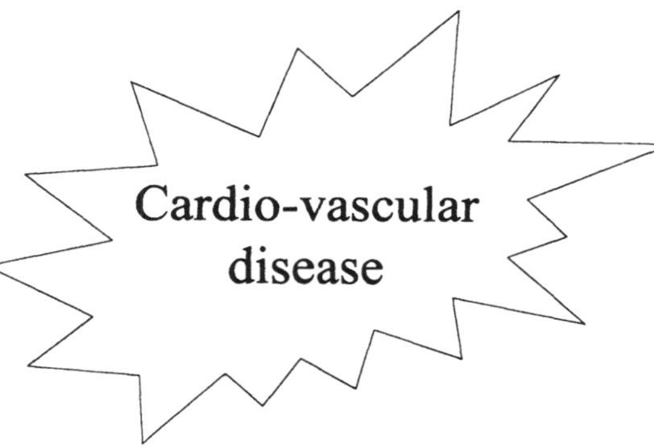

skeletal problems

Fatigue

Handout for homework exercise

- 1. Choose a person from around you such as a child, parent, neighbour, friend or other person and tell them that you are attending a readjustment meeting for your hearing problem
- 2. Try to explain to this person something of what you learnt about the effects of hearing loss in the lives of Deafened people

- To help you with the explanations, you can use the handouts from the programme

Hearing tactics: a restaurant

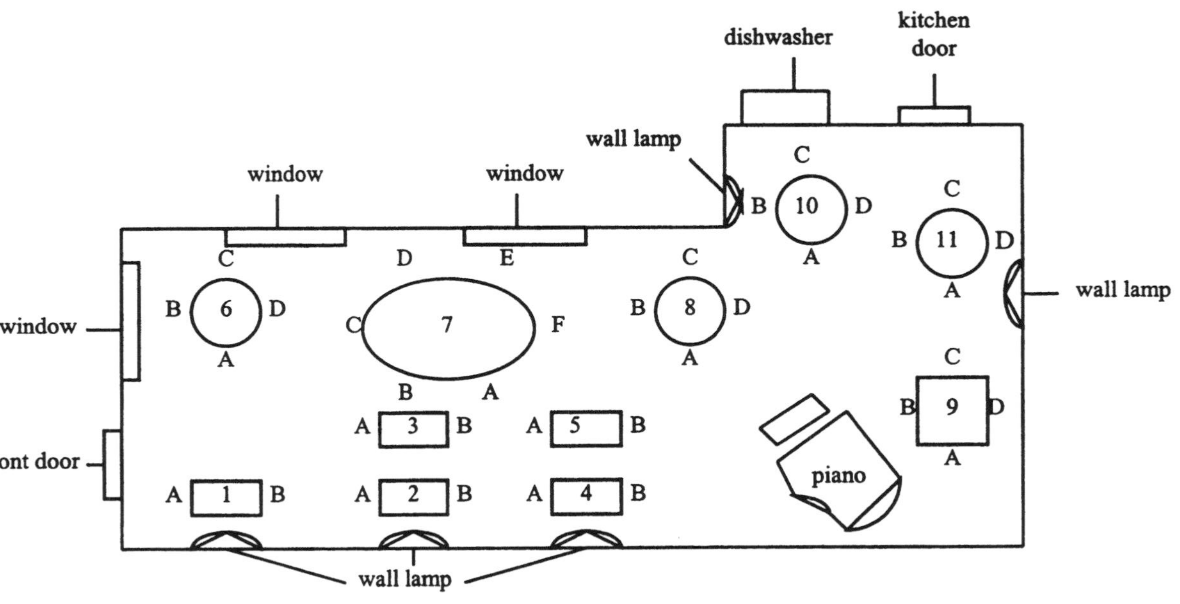

Source: adapted from Kaplan, Bally and Garrestson (1985).

Responding to challenging situations 1 – the doctor's waiting room

- You have been sitting in your doctor's waiting room for nearly an hour past your appointment time. People who have arrived after you have been seen by your doctor. The receptionist at the desk seems to be unaware of your lengthy wait. You decide to:
- Passive____
- ____

- Aggressive:______________________________________
- ____

- Assertive:_______________________________________
- ____

Source: adapted from an original design by Christopher Lind, Victorian Hear Service – used with permission.

Choosing a holiday – people with hearing loss

- You and your partner have decided to purchase a holiday. You've been looking at brochures for a while now and have finally decided on a place you would like to go to. You go to visit a travel agent to get more information about your chosen destination and to ask about special offers and prices. As the travel agent begins to answer your questions he is distracted by some other activity in the agency and begins to turn away as he answers you. Consequently, you found it difficult to follow the information you were given.

Choosing a holiday – partners

- You and your partner have decided to purchase a holiday. You've been looking at brochures for a while now and have finally decided on a place you would like to go to. You go to visit a travel agent to get more information about your chosen destination and to ask about special offers and prices. As the travel agent begins to answer your questions he is distracted by some other activity in the agency and begins to turn away as he answers you. Consequently, your partner found it difficult to follow the information you were given.

Marion's dinner party – handout for people with hearing loss

Marion, your partner's cousin, likes entertaining a lot. It will soon be her husband's birthday and she wants to make the most of this and organize a big celebratory dinner. And of course she invites you and your partner. You arrive at Marion's, she introduces you to the people you don't know and soon afterwards invites you to go to the dinner. As she has decided to mix everyone up, she assigns a place for you away from your partner. You find yourself three places away, between Marion and someone you don't know. Marion wanted to create a good atmosphere, so she has subdued lights and has background music playing on their new compact disc player. To decorate the table she has candles and a large bouquet of flowers, which just happens to be in front of your place. The meal is good, the beer is cold and the wine excellent. Everyone is having a good time, things are warming up and everyone seems to be talking at once. There are some who have had a fair bit to drink and they talk more quickly and less distinctively than at the start of the evening. Marion, who knows you have difficulty hearing tries to say something to you, speaking very slowly and exaggerating her pronunciation; the person next to you looks at her and seems to wonder what is going on. You hasten to change the subject…

Marion's dinner party – handout for partners

Marion, your cousin, likes entertaining a lot. It will soon be her husband's birthday and she wants to make the most of this and organize a big celebratory dinner. And of course she invites you and your partner. You arrive at Marion's, she introduces you to the people you don't know and soon afterwards invites you to go to the dinner. As she had decided to mix everyone up, she assigns a place for you away from your partner. You find yourself three places away, and your partner is between Marion and someone you don't know. Marion wanted to create a good atmosphere, so she has subdued lights and has background music playing on their new compact disc player. To decorate the table she has candles and a large bouquet of flowers, which just happens to be in front of your partner. The meal is good, the beer is cold and the wine excellent. Everyone is having a good time, things are warming up and everyone seems to be talking at once. There are some who have had a fair bit to drink and they talk more quickly and less distinctively than at the start of the evening. Marion, who knows your partner has difficulty hearing tries to say something to your partner, speaking very slowly and exaggerating her pronunciation; the person next to your partner looks at her and seems to wonder what is going on. Your partner hastens to change the subject…

Marion's dinner party

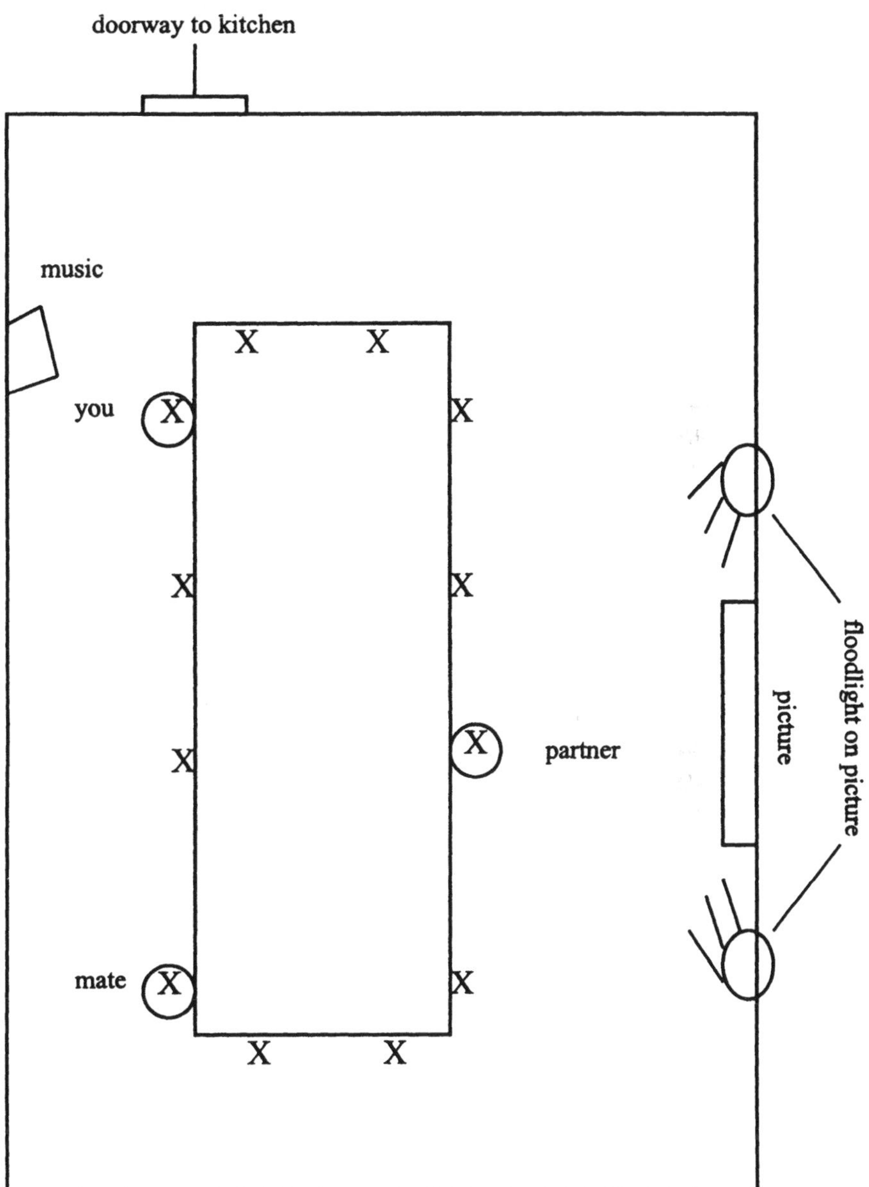

Relaxation exercise

- Focus on point 1" below navel in the middle of your body
- Breathe deeply
- Expand lower abdomen as you breathe in
- Flatten abdomen as you breathe out
- Do for 10–20 minutes

Responding to challenging situations 2 – making an appointment at the dentist

- You have just come out of your appointment with the dentist and you need to make a new time. Your ask the receptionist for a time. She says something to you, but you're not sure what it was she said.
- Passive____
- ____

- Aggressive:____
- ____

- Assertive:____
- ____

Source: adapted from an original design by Christopher Lind, Victorian Hear Service – used with permission.

Responding to challenging situations 3 – at the bank

- You find yourself waiting in line at a local bank. In this bank the tellers stand behind bullet-proof glass. Each customer window is fitted with a microphone system and some have loops fitted. However, the staff rarely use any of the technology provided. In consequence, it is very difficult to communicate with the bank's staff.

- What 'I' statement could you make here to assert your communication needs with the bank?

Source: adapted from an original design by Christopher Lind, Victorian Hear Service – used with permission.

Taking responsibility – people with hearing loss

- You and your partner are attending the doctors to find out the results of some tests you have had and to discuss a management plan for your health. The doctor is running late and appears flustered. You have had to wait a couple of months to see this doctor. The medical condition has been worrying you and you realise this is an important opportunity to sort things out. You are finding it difficult to follow the information you are being given.

Taking responsibility – partners

- You and your partner are attending the doctors to find out the results of some tests your partner has had and to discuss a management plan for your partner's health. The doctor is running late and appears flustered. You have had to wait a couple of months to see this doctor. The medical condition has been worrying your partner and you realise this is an important opportunity to sort things out. Your partner is finding it difficult to follow the information they are being given.

Managing at work

- You work in a small office and regularly take material into your supervisor for discussion. The supervisor has a small office and you usually sit opposite her when you go in to see her. Although the supervisor has been trained in communicating with you, she is not very sympathetic to your needs and quickly gets impatient with you. On this occasion, you take an important piece of work into the supervisor that you have been working on for some time. You are keen to impress on the supervisor how well you've done with this project. The supervisor looks at it, starts to write on what you have done and makes comments to you about it. Unfortunately, you missed most of what she said as she was looking down as she spoke, and she had her hand over her head (as if to concentrate). To make matters worse, the photocopy machine, which is just outside the door, was running, making it more difficult for you to hear. The supervisor looks up at you (somewhat sternly) as though she were waiting for you to respond to whatever it was she said.

Personal contract

Personal contract

From now until the next meeting I intend to:

- explain to people that I have a hearing problem
- make requests in keeping with my hearing problem
- investigate and/or get myself a new telephone with volume control
- investigate and/or get myself a TV aid
- investigate hearing aids
- investigate and/or get myself a cochlear implant/use my accessories
- investigate/get myself/use accessories that go with my cochlear implant speech processor
- look more at people when I'm listening to them
- Other (please say what)....................................
-
- Signed.................................
- Date...................................

Sample follow-up letter that may be used to invite participants to follow-up meeting

Sample follow-up letter

Hello everyone,
You will remember recently doing a workshop with me on living with Hearing Loss. At this meeting, as well as looking at the impact of hearing loss in our lives, we saw several ways to make life easier with our hearing problems.

For example, we saw that by planning ahead or being assertive, one could make hearing in difficult places more manageable. You will also have realized that there are non-technical means to help oneself, in particular, in group meetings or in outings. We all know the usual tactics for improving communication like asking people to talk more slowly, repeating, talking face to face, and reducing background noise. In the group the key to success was identified as being confident and assertive and being prepared to plan ahead to minimize the chance of problems arising. Through planning and being assertive we can make communicating easier and we can lessen stress by using relaxation.

It's been 3 months since we met and it's time for a brief follow-up meeting. The purpose of the meeting is to see where you are now, to find out what you've been doing and to see if there is anything else we can do to support you as you move on to manage your everyday communication needs. As well, we would like some feedback on what you thought of the workshop and how it can be improved.

Looking forward to seeing you again at (place, time, date)

Scales

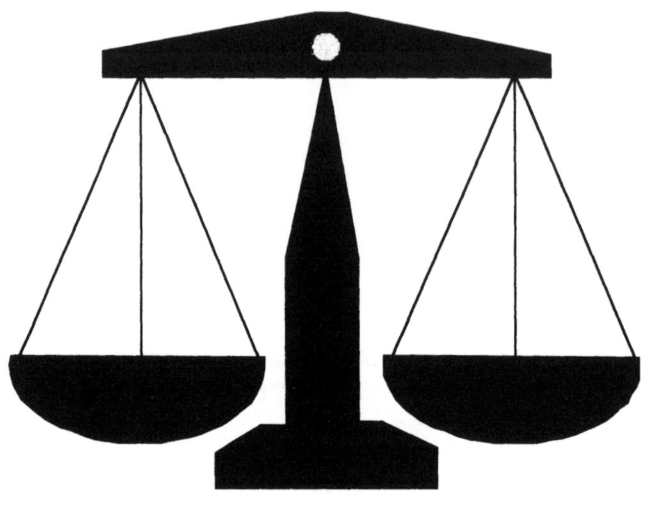

Index

ableism 6, 11, 45–6, 53
Access 2000 kits 149, 151, 188–9
acupuncture 93, 168
age 25, 30, 61, 64, 66, 95, 126
  early onset of deafness 26–9, 31
  employment 37–9, 42, 132–5
  later onset of deafness 31–6
aggression 91, 172, 174–5, 186
aidable thresholds 25–6
alcohol 84, 86, 158, 182, 216–17, 231–2
anomie 14–15, 17–19, 23
aromatherapy 93, 169
assertiveness 12, 73, 77, 91–2, 173–5, 187–8
  CMP 101
  communcation skills programme 151, 172–5, 186–8, 192–3, 195, 241
  contested identity 56
  developing communication skills 85, 88–90
  structuring interventions 115, 121, 124
Assessment of Quality of Life 95
assistive listening devices 11, 76, 78, 115, 180–1
  assertiveness 92
  communication skills programme 150–2, 180–1, 188
  developing communication skills 88
audiograms 84, 151, 155–6
audiologists 29, 76, 106
  attitudes to cochlear implants 61–4, 67
Australian Hearing Services 76
avoidance behaviours 15–16

background noise 195, 216–17, 219, 241
  developing communication skills 82, 84, 88
  employment 137
  parties 158–9, 161, 182, 231–2
  restaurants 6–7
banks 13–14, 187, 236
barbecue party 84, 86, 147, 151, 156–61, 162, 182
  handouts 215–17
Battelle Institute 200
bio-mechanical model 7, 52
Birmingham Centre for Deafened Adults 93
birthday parties 151, 156–61, 196

case histories 98–9
chiropractors 93, 168
closure 117, 129–30
cochlear implants 3, 6, 11, 72, 76, 78, 96–100
  assessment 117–22
  CMP 100–5, 112
  communication skills programme 147–98

contested identity 43, 48, 53, 55, 56–7
decision-making 120–3
eligibility 62–5, 66–7, 68
employment 37–40, 64–6, 68, 96, 98, 109, 131–8, 143
everyday barriers 61–71
everyday benefits 139–43
expectations 70, 96–102, 105–7, 108–11, 115–17, 121–6
helping relationship 96
intensive rehabilitation 123–7
maintenance and closure 129–30
methodological issues 199–200
ongoing support 127–9
onset of deafness 24, 26, 37–40, 61, 64, 68, 140
practical limitations 109–10
reconciling reality 107–9
structuring interventions 115–24
switch-on 105–7, 109, 123–4, 126
Cochlear Limited 200
Code-Muller Protocols (CMP) 100–5, 111, 112–14
evaluating outcomes 95
MAUT 103–5
structuring interventions 122–3, 126
coherency 22, 27–8, 30, 33–6, 89
contested identity 44, 50, 52
communication skills 56, 73–6, 79–80, 94, 101
development 81–90
everyday benefits of cochlear implants 139, 140–3
handouts 212–42
programme 147–98
rules for workshop 153, 212
structuring interventions 115, 121, 126
communicative action 35–6
complementary and alternative therapies 69, 76, 93
confidence 10, 75, 77, 88, 94–5, 121, 126
cochlear implants 68, 70, 109, 141–2
communication skills programme 148, 154, 195, 197
evaluating outcomes 95
formation of the self 12, 15
handouts 214, 241
identity 18, 21
congruence 81, 102, 103, 114
continuity 22, 81, 89
contested identity 44–5, 52
onset of deafness 25, 27–8, 30, 33, 35–6
contracts 122–3, 129, 192–3, 240
costs and funding 62–3, 65, 68, 95, 110
counselling 20, 36, 51, 93
CMP 100–3, 122–3, 126
cochlear implants 66, 98–102, 108–9, 111, 126
structuring interventions 115–16, 119, 121–3, 126
CPHI 95
CRS Australia 133

deep breathing exercises 184–5, 192, 234
dentists 186, 235
depression 27, 32
CMP 100, 103–5, 112–13
dinner parties 151, 182–3, 231–3
disability pensions 41
discrimination 6–7, 10, 42, 45–6, 56, 187
divestment 54
doctors 173–5, 189–91, 228, 237–8
doorbells 50, 98, 108, 140
flashing lights 51, 98, 108
duration of deafness 64, 66–8, 133–4

earnings and income 6, 39–40, 42, 57, 72, 95
cochlear implants 65–6, 96, 129
disability pensions 41
employment outcomes 131–2, 136, 138
education 6, 20, 26–9, 97, 120, 200
contested identity 49, 53
employment 37–42, 133–4
evaluating outcomes 95
onset of deafness 25, 26–9, 31, 37–42
qualifications 37–9, 133
embarrassment 16, 19, 175
CMP 100–5, 112–13
developing communication skills 85–7, 90
employment 6, 36–42, 72, 79, 95, 126–7, 200
CMP 100, 103–5, 112–13

cochlear implants 37–40, 64–6, 68, 96, 98, 109, 131–8, 143
communication skills programme 151, 191–2, 197, 239
contested identity 49, 53, 57
enhancing outcomes 131–8
evaluating outcomes 95
formation of the self 12
independence 8
onset of deafness 25, 30–2, 34, 36–42
promotion 12, 42, 137, 143
qualifications 37–9
structuring interventions 120, 121, 126–7, 128–9
workforce participation rate 38, 42
environmental sounds 79, 108, 111, 140
EuroQol 95
expectations 115–17, 121–6, 136
CMP 100–2
cochlear implants 70, 96–102, 105–7, 108–11, 115–17, 121–6

fear 70, 86
formation of the self 15–16, 18
follow-up to workshop 151, 194–8, 241
frustration 159, 220
CMP 100–5, 112–13

general practitioners 62–3
Glasgow Hearing Benefit Inventory 95
guilt 11, 16, 48, 98, 108, 159, 220

health 6, 72, 79, 93, 95, 96, 120
employment 131
Hear Service Programme 147
hearing aids 3, 6, 11, 72, 76, 78
contested identity 43, 47–8, 50–1, 53
communication skills programme 149, 175, 178, 180, 193, 240
onset of deafness 24, 26
structuring interventions 122
hearing handicap questionnaire 121, 122
Hearing Help cards 149, 188–9, 197
Hearing and Listening Skills Programme 147
hearing tactics 48, 72–4, 76, 85, 89–90, 172
heuristics 15, 90
hobbies 31, 34, 129, 169
CMP 100, 102–5, 112–13
holidays 176–8, 229–30
homeopathy 93
homework exercise 151, 170, 171, 226
hook-up 105–7, 123–4, 126

I statements 87–90, 91
communication skills programme 153, 159, 163, 172–3, 175, 182, 187, 192
handouts 212, 218, 236
ice breakers 148, 196
identity 10, 17–23, 43–57, 73, 88, 94, 148
awareness exercise 151, 180
decision-making 121
formation of the self 12, 15
later onset of deafness 31, 34–5
independence 7, 8–9, 70, 126–7, 141, 176
CMP 100, 103–5, 112–13
insurers 41, 46, 62, 65, 68, 95
integrated case management 116–18
isolation 16, 18, 21, 73, 85
cochlear implants 98, 140
identity 18, 21, 50
onset of deafness 27, 29, 34

lighting 84–5, 150, 158–9, 161, 182
handouts 216–17, 219, 231–2
Link Centre for Deafened Adults 56, 76, 92, 93
lip-reading 27–9, 30, 33–4, 76, 88
cochlear implants 65–6, 108–9, 111, 115, 142
contested identity 48–51, 53, 55
employment 40, 137

maintenance 117, 127, 129–30
making new friends 100, 102, 103–5, 112–13
marginalization 18, 69, 73, 91
contested identity 47–8, 50, 52–3, 56–7
onset of deafness 28, 31, 33, 35
massage 93, 169
Mater Adult Cochlear Implant Programme 133–6

medical model of disability 7–8, 10, 11, 20
contested identity 43–4, 48
motivation 69, 98, 115, 120, 123
Multiple Attribute Utility Technique (MAUT) 103–5, 113

National Acoustic Laboratory 76
normalness and normalization 5–7, 12, 14
contested identity 45–6, 48–9
onset of deafness 27–8, 31, 34

ongoing support 117, 127–9
onset of deafness 12, 24–42, 72, 90, 120
cochlear implants 24, 26, 37–40, 61, 64, 68, 140
early 2609, 31
employment 25, 30–2, 34, 36–42
gradual 31, 34, 37, 140
identity 17, 23, 43, 45–7, 56–7
later 31–6
sudden 29–31, 32, 33, 68, 119

paging systems 30, 37
passivity 91, 172, 174–5, 186
peer support 51, 53–4
Perceptual Congruence Quotient (PCQ) 102, 114
phonocentricism 6, 13–14, 20–1, 35, 52
planning ahead 88, 92, 172, 195, 241
pretend deaf people 51
problem exploration 80, 84–6, 89, 148
problem identification 80, 81–4, 86, 94, 148
problem resolution 76–7, 79, 87–90, 92, 94, 116
communication skills programme 148, 191
structuring interventions 121
psychotherapy 83, 93, 99

Queensland Cochlear Implant Clinic 147

referrals 121, 126–7, 130
cochlear implants 62–4, 66–8
employment 126–7, 132–3, 135–6
psychotherapy 83, 99
relaxation 94

relaxation 88, 90, 93–4, 128–9
communication skills programme 148, 151, 166–9, 171, 175, 184–5, 192–3, 195, 197
exercises 151, 169, 184–5, 192, 234
handouts 218, 234, 241
remaking oneself 5, 11, 23, 24, 47, 52, 96
decision-making 121
maintenance and closure 129
repetition 13, 32, 82
cochlear implants 109, 141
communication skills programme 159, 177, 191, 195, 220
restaurants 6–8, 73, 86, 88, 91–2
communication skills programme 147, 151, 171–3, 181
handout 227
role-playing 91, 172–3, 175, 187, 191–2
rubella 74

safety of cochlear implants 66
scoping interviews 119–20, 122
self-esteem 10, 105, 129, 142
identity 18–19, 21
shame 10–11, 16–18, 87, 90
identity 18–19, 21, 46–8
sign language 3, 12, 61, 69, 118, 140–1
contested identity 46, 50–1, 53
onset of deafness 27–8, 30
Sintonen 15d 95
social connectedness 139, 140
social model of disability 7–8, 9, 11
socialization 100, 103–5, 112–13
speaking to strangers 100, 103–5, 112–13
stigmatization 45, 46, 48, 73
developing communication skills 85, 87, 89
stress 13–16, 32, 72–3, 76, 93, 108, 162–9
assertiveness 91
cochlear implants 70, 106, 142
communication skills programme 161, 162–9, 171–3, 191, 195, 197
developing communication skills 83, 85
handouts 221–5, 241
identity 19–20, 50–2
structuring interventions 118, 120, 129

technologies of the self 4, 22, 199
telephone typewriters (TTYs) 37, 51, 181
telephone use 154, 181, 193, 214, 240
  cochlear implants 53, 65, 107, 108, 140, 141
  employment 30, 37, 40, 49, 133
tragedy model of disability 7–8, 10, 20, 36

unfair hearing test 84, 137
University of Sydney 93

water sports 65

9 781861 562159

Made in the USA
Lexington, KY
10 May 2012